Intermitter

for Women over 50

The Ultimate Step-by-Step Guide for Losing Weight Rapidly, Burning Fat and Improving the Quality of Life

SANDRA NEEL

Your Free Gift

As a way of saying thanks for your purchase, to our readers we offer as a gift a printable recipe book, to download for free: "Cookbook Journal", a diary in which to keep track of all your culinary inventions, assigning each one an evaluation, the difficulty of execution and much more.

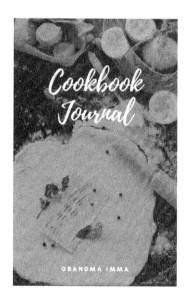

Click this link to free download
https://dl.bookfunnel.com/i3sq7ljm6z

Table of Contents

Introduction

Intermittent Fasting (IF) is one of the most successful health and wellness phenomena in the world right now. It is being used by people to lose weight, boost their fitness, and improve their lifestyles.

Many types of research have shown that it may have a significant impact on the body and brain and that it can also help you live longer. Intermittent fasting is a method of eating, not a diet. It's a method of planning your foods so that you get the best bang for your buck. Intermittent fasting does not change your eating habits; however, it changes the timing of your meals.

Most importantly, it's a smart way to get lean without being on a fad diet or severely restricting your calorie intake. In reality, when you first start intermittent fasting, you'll try to maintain your calorie intake constant. (Most people consume larger meals in a shorter period of time.) Intermittent fasting is often a healthy way to maintain muscle strength when losing weight.

Having said that, the main motivation for people to pursue intermittent fasting is to lose weight. In a moment, we will discuss how intermittent fasting helps you lose weight.

And most notably, since it takes relatively little behavior change, intermittent fasting is one of the best methods we have for losing weight and maintaining a healthy weight. This is a positive thing because it implies intermittent fasting falls under the category of "easy enough to perform, but significant enough to make a difference."

Intermittent fasting can be done in various ways, but they both include selecting regular eating and fasting times. For example, you might consider eating just for eight hours a day and fasting for the rest of the day. Alternatively, you might decide to eat just one food a day, two days a week. There are a variety of intermittent fasting routines to choose from.

According to Mattson, the body's sugar stores are exhausted after hours without food, and it begins to burn fat. This is referred to as metabolic switching by him.

"Most Americans eat in their waking hours, but intermittent fasting is in comparison to their usual eating pattern," Mattson adds. "If somebody eats three meals a day with treats and doesn't exercise, they're living on some calories and then not burning the fat stores any time they eat."

Intermittent fasting operates by extending the time from when the body burns off the calories from your last meal and starts burning fat.

To understand how IF contributes to fat loss, we must first understand the distinction between the fed and fasted state.

When the body digests and absorbs food, this is in a fed state. The fed condition usually begins when you start feeding and lasts 3 to 5 hours as your body digest and consumes the food you just consumed. Since your insulin levels are higher while you're in the fed state, it's difficult for your body to burn fat.

During that time period, the body enters a condition recognized as the post-absorptive state, that is just a fancy way of suggesting that it isn't processing a meal. The post-absorptive condition continues before you reach the fasted state, which is 8 to 12 hrs after your last meal. Since your insulin levels are low, it is much simpler for your body to lose fat while you have fasted.

When you're fasting, your body has the ability to burn fat that was previously inaccessible.

Our bodies are rarely in this fat-burning condition, and we don't reach the fasted state till 12 hours after our last meal. This is one of the explanations that many people who begin intermittent fasting lose weight without changing their diet, amount of food consumed, or frequency of exercise. Fasting induces a fat-burning condition in your body that you seldom achieve with a regular feeding schedule.

Why do people fast?

Although weight loss is one of the advantages of intermittent fasting, it is not the same as dieting. It's an eating plan with long-term benefits, including controlling insulin levels, preventing diabetes, and even helping you maintain a healthier weight.

This may go against what you have learned in the past regarding eating frequency. Your body would not go into "starvation mode" if you skip a meal. And, while there's nothing wrong with consuming breakfast, there are several advantages of taking a long break between meals.

Chapter: 1 Intermittent Fasting

In recent years, intermittent fasting has increased in popularity.

Intermittent fasting, unlike most diets, relies on what to eat by adding daily short-term fasts into the schedule.

This eating style can assist you in consuming fewer calories, losing weight, and reducing your risk of developing diabetes and heart disease.

On the other hand, intermittent fasting could not be as effective for women as it is for men, according to a collection of studies. As a result, women may need to take a different approach.

For women, here's a step-by-step guide to intermittent fasting.

1.1 What Is Intermittent Fasting?

Intermittent fasting is an eating cycle under which you alternate between eating and fasting periods. It does not specify the foods should be consumed, but rather when they should be consumed. There are a variety of intermittent fasting strategies available, many of which divide the day or week into eating and fasting times. The majority of people still "fast" while sleeping every day. Trying to extend the fast can be an easy way to practice intermittent fasting. Skip breakfast, eat the first lunch at midday, and the last meal at 8 p.m. to do this. Then you're basically fasting for 16 hours a day, with an 8-hour eating window. The 16/8 approach is the most widely used type of intermittent fasting.

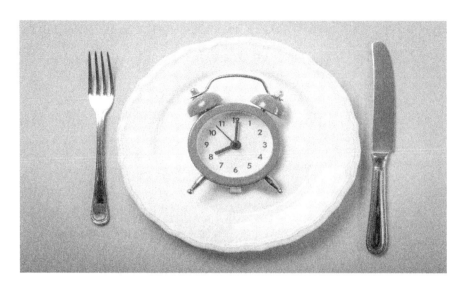

Intermittent fasting is really very easy, despite popular belief. During a fast, several people report feeling healthier and getting more energy. Hunger is normally not a challenge, but it may be at the beginning when the body adjusts to not eating for long periods of time. During the fasting time, no food is permitted, although water, coffee, tea, and other non-caloric drinks are permitted. During the fasting time, certain types of intermittent fasting provide for limited quantities of low-calorie foods. Taking vitamins when fasting is normally permitted as long as they provide no calories.

1.2 How Does It Affect the Hormones and Cells?

On a cellular and molecular basis, when you fast, many things happen in your body. Your body, for example, changes hormone levels to allow retained body fat more available.

Essential repair steps and gene expression changes are often initiated by your cells. When you fast, your body undergoes the following changes:

- **Human Growth Hormone:** Growth hormone levels increase, often by as many as 5-fold. This has a number of advantages, including weight loss and muscle gain.

- **Cellular repair:** When you fast, your cells begin to repair themselves. Autophagy is a process in which cells ingest and destroy old and inactive proteins that have accumulated within them.

- **Insulin:** Insulin sensitivity increases and insulin levels decrease significantly. Insulin levels that are lower allow stored body fat more available.

- **Gene expression:** There are several variations in gene regulation that are linked to survival and disease resistance.

Intermittent fasting's health advantages are due to improvements in hormone levels, cell structure, and gene expression.

1.3 Highly Effective Weight-Loss Tool

The most popular cause for people to attempt intermittent fasting is to lose weight. Intermittent fasting will automatically reduce the calorie consumption by pushing you to consume less meals.

Intermittent fasting often alters hormone levels, which helps weight reduction. It raises the production of the burn fat hormone norepinephrine in addition to reducing insulin and raising growth hormone levels (noradrenaline).

Short-term fasting can increase your metabolism by 3.6 to 14 percent as a result of these hormonal changes.

Intermittent fasting induces weight reduction by altering all aspects of the calorie spectrum by assisting you in eating less and burning further calories. Intermittent fasting has been shown in studies to be a very effective weight-loss technique.

This eating pattern will result in 3 to 8 percent weight loss over 3 to 24 weeks, according to a 2014 analysis report, which is a large amount as compared to other weight loss studies.

People have lost 4 to 7 percent of their waist circumference, showing a substantial loss of unhealthy belly fat that develops around the organs and induces illness, according to the same report.

In another analysis, intermittent fasting was shown to induce less muscle weakness than the more common form of constant calorie restriction.

Bear in mind, though, that the biggest explanation for its popularity is that it allows you to gain less calories, and you do not lose much weight if you binge and consume more through your feeding hours.

1.4 How Does It Work?

It can be strange that merely changing your eating schedule will help you lose weight. About this, our bodies adapt to fasting in a positive way. When your body goes into fasting mode, your fat reserves are called upon to be used as food, allowing you to consume fat for energy.

Of course, just because you aren't fasting doesn't suggest you should eat whatever you want. To get the best outcomes, eat nutritious whole grains, lean proteins and unrefined carbohydrates. Keep in mind that calorie-free beverages like tea, black coffee and water should be consumed during fasting times. You might also note that you are feeding more slowly and for greater enjoyment.

You won't have to starve yourself if you practice intermittent fasting, also known as IF. It also doesn't owe you permission to eat a bunch of fatty food while you aren't fasting. Instead of consuming meals and treats during the day, you feed over a set period of time.

The majority of people adhere to an IF pattern that allows them to fast for 12 to 16 hours a day. They enjoy regular meals and treats the majority of the day. Since most people sleep for around eight hours during their fasting hours, sticking to this feeding window isn't as difficult as it sounds. You're often allowed to consume zero-calorie drinks like water, tea, & coffee. Quick Bars should also be eaten in between meals to keep the fast going.

For the strongest intermittent fasting outcomes, build an eating routine that works for you. Consider the following example:

- **12-hour fasts:** If you follow a 12-hour fast, you will miss breakfast and snacks at lunchtime. You might eat an early supper and skip evening snacks if you want to eat your morning lunch. A 12-12 quick is relatively simple to maintain for most older women.

- **16-hour fasts:** A 16-8 IF timetable can yield faster results. Within an 8-hour span, most people prefer to eat two meals and a snack or two. For example, the eating timeframe may be fixed between noon and 8 p.m. or between 8 a.m. and 4 p.m.

- **5-2 routine:** You might not be able to stick to a restricted eating schedule every day. Another choice is to follow a 12- or 16-hour quick for five days and then rest for two days. For example, you might do intermittent fasting throughout the week and eat regularly on the weekends.

- **Fasting any other day:** Another choice is to eat very little calories on alternating days. For instance, you might restrict your calories to under 500 calories one day and then eat normally the next. It's worth noting that regular IF fasts never necessitate calorie restrictions that low.

You'll have the strongest effects from this diet if you stick to it. Around the same period, on rare days, you should certainly take a break from this type of eating routine. You should try different types of intermittent fasting to see which one is well for you. Many people begin their IF journey with the 12-12 plan and then move to the 16-8 plan. After that, continue to adhere to the schedule as accurately as possible.

1.5 Science behind Intermittent Fasting

There's still some science at work here, in the form of your body's HGH development. Until we get into that, let me clarify why this is the case. Our bodies generate insulin to preserve glucose from carbohydrates for subsequent use while we feed. We live in a world where much of our meals are routine, and we are constantly bombarded with foods that are high in sugar and fat. This places us in an anabolic situation, which means we're still gaining weight. Food glucose is processed as fat, resulting in weight gain. Intermittent fasting effectively reverses this mechanism, allowing our cells to use the glucose that has been processed in our cells for energy. Weight loss occurs as cells reach a catabolic (breaking down) state. HGH is generated in reaction to the body's need for glucose, but while we consume often, our HGH output is suppressed because we are consuming glucose from outside sources. HGH is a hormone that controls metabolism and has many benefits for muscle regeneration and fat burning. Fasting for short periods of time has been shown to increase HGH productivity by up to 5 times.

1.6 Intermittent Fasting for Longevity

Another part of intermittent fasting that I find intriguing and ground-breaking (forgive the expression) is its anti-aging efficacy and the benefits it brings to longevity. This is largely accomplished by autophagy, which is the body's normal means of destroying weakened cells and replacing them with fresh, stable ones. It's similar to recycling. This is very exciting in terms of longevity. A natural, natural way to replace old cells and switch back the clock with the development of new ones. Autophagy is a natural process that our ancestors instilled in us to provide nutrition to the body (self-eating). Of course, this won't continue forever, but since you'll be eating all day, the body won't be able to sustain it. When our cells get stressed, intermittent fasting increases autophagy. Autophagy is activated to defend and replenish the body. This actually prolongs our lives. I like listening to Dr. (whatshisname?) lecture because he has tested all of these hypotheses on rats. What he's discovered is incredible. He was able to demonstrate confidently that CR would extend the lifetime of rats by 30%. There are no drugs or medicines involved, only a common trick that we can all use.

1.7 Is Intermittent Fasting Healthy?

Is overnight fasting a healthy way to eat? Remember that you can just fast for 12 to 16 hours at a time, not for days. You also have a lot of time to eat a delicious and nutritious meal. Of course, certain older women may need regular eating due to metabolic diseases or drug guidelines. Under any scenario, you can talk to the doctor about your dietary patterns before implementing any changes.

Although it isn't actually fasting, some physicians claim that allowing easy-to-digest foods like whole fruit and during the fasting, the window has health benefits. Modifications like this will also provide a much-needed break for the digestive and metabolic systems. For example, the famous weight-loss book "Fit for Life" recommended consuming just fruit after supper & before lunch.

In reality, according to the writers of this novel, they had patients who just modified their eating patterns by fasting for 12 to 16 hours per day. They didn't obey the rest of the diet's guidelines or count calories, but they also shed weight and improved their fitness. This technique may have failed largely because dieters substituted fast food with whole foods. In either scenario, participants considered this dietary modification to be beneficial and simple to implement. Traditionalists won't term this fasting, so it's good to remember that if you can't go without eating for many hours at a time, you may have some choices.

1.8 Who should not try for Intermittent Fasting?

Intermittent fasting isn't suitable for anyone. Before starting every new diet, even one that has been shown to be beneficial, you should still consult a doctor. If you belong to one of the following parties, you can stop it:

- Diabetes patients and others with other blood sugar issues.

- Children under the age of eighteen.

- People who have had an eating disorder in the past

- Women who are pregnant or breastfeeding.

1.9 How to Get Started with Intermittent Fasting?

Intermittent fasting includes cycling between eating and fasting periods. People can find it hard at first to eat just for a brief period of time per day or to switch between eating and not eating days. This chapter describes advice about how to get started fasting, such as setting personal goals, preparing menus, and determining calorie requirements.

Intermittent fasting is a common strategy for achieving the following goals:

- Get their lives easier.

- Weight loss.

- Minimize the symptoms of aging, and increase their physical health and well-being.

Fasting is generally suitable for most fit, well-nourished people, although it might not be sufficient for those with medical conditions. The following tips are intended to assist those who are ready to begin fasting in making it as simple and successful as possible.

1. Identify your personal goals

2. Pick the method

3. Figure out caloric needs

4. Figure out a meal plan

5. Make the calories count

Now, we discuss these tips step by step;

1. Identify Your Personal Goals

A person who begins intermittent fasting usually has a specific target in mind. That may be for weight loss, better physical health, or better metabolic function. A person's overall objective can help them in determining the best fasting approach and calculating how much calories and nutrients they need.

2. Select the Method

When it comes to fasting for health benefits, there are four options to consider. An individual should choose the plan that best suits their needs and that they believe they will be able to stick with.

Before attempting a new fasting method, an individual can usually stay with one for a month or longer to see how it works for them. Before starting any fasting process, someone with a medical condition can consult their doctor.

When choosing a method, keep in mind that you don't have to consume a particular quantity or type of food or skip certain foods entirely. An individual is free to consume whatever they want. During the feeding times, though, it is a smart idea to consume a balanced, high-fiber, vegetable-rich diet to achieve health and weight loss targets.

On eating days, overindulging in unhealthy foods will damage your health. On fast days, it's often important to consume plenty of water or other low-calorie drinks.

- **Eat Stop Eat**

Eat Stop Eat was created by Brad Pilon, and it is a fasting process that entails not eating for 24 hours twice a week. It makes no difference how many days an individual fasts or when they begin. The only stipulation is that fasting must be done for at least 24 hours and on non-consecutive days.

People who go without eating for more than 24 hours are likely to get really hungry. Eat Stop Eat might not be the right way for people who are new to fasting.

- **Warrior Diet**

The Warrior Diet, created by Ori Hofmekler, involves consuming very little for 20 hours per day. In the remaining four hours, individual fasting in this manner eats all of their typical food intakes.

Eating a whole day's worth of food in such a brief period of time will disturb a person's stomach. This is the most intense fasting technique, and like Eat Stop Eat, it is not recommended for someone who is new to fasting.

- **Leangains**

Leangains was founded by Martin Berkhan for weightlifters, but it has since gained popularity among some other persons involved in fasting. Fasting for Leangains is much shorter than it is for Eat Stop Eat & the Warrior Diet.

Males who prefer the Leangains process, for example, will fast for 16 hours and then consume anything they desire for the remaining 8 hours. Females fast for 14 hours and then consume whatever they want for the next 10 hours.

During the fast, one must prohibit from consuming some food but can consume as many non-calorie drinks as desired.

- **5:2 process of alternate-day fasting**

To increase cholesterol, blood sugar, and weight reduction, certain people fast on alternating days. On the 5:2 diet, a person consumes 500 to 600 calories on two non-consecutive days per week.

Some alternate-day fasting plans have a third fasting day each week. A person consumes just the number of calories they burn throughout the day for the rest of the week. This results in a calorie deficit over time, allowing the individual to lose weight.

3. Figure out Caloric Needs

When fasting, there are no food limits, but calories must always be counted.

People who choose to lose weight would build a calorie shortage, which implies they must gain fewer calories than they consume. Many that want to gain weight would eat more calories than they consume.

There are several resources available to assist a person in calculating their caloric requirements and determining how much calories they must eat per day to gain or lose weight. An individual may also seek advice from a healthcare professional or a dietitian on how much calories they need.

4. Figure out a Meal Plan

A person who is trying to lose or gain weight can feel that planning their meals for the day or week is beneficial.

Meal preparation does not have to be conservative. It takes into consideration calorie consumption as well as ensuring the right foods are used in the diet.

Meal preparation has a number of advantages, including assisting with calorie counting and ensuring that an individual has the requisite food on hand for preparing recipes, fast dinners, and snacks.

5. Make the Calories Needs

Calories aren't always made equal. Since these fasting practices do not indicate how much calories an individual can consume when fasting, the nutritional content of the food must be considered.

In general, nutrient-dense food, or meals with a large number of nutrients per calorie, should be consumed. Even if a person does not have to completely avoid fast food, they can also eat it in moderation and concentrate on healthier alternatives to gain the most rewards.

Chapter: 2 Types of Intermittent Fasting

There are a lot of various ways to do intermittent fasting, which is fantastic. If this is something you are interested in, you may choose the kind that better suits the needs, increasing your chances of success. Here are seven of them:

1. 5:2 Fasting

2. Time-Restricted Fasting

3. Overnight Fasting

4. Eat Stop Eat

5. Whole-Day Fasting

6. Alternate-Day Fasting

7. Choose-Your-Day Fasting

The above seven types of intermittent fasting are explained step by step.

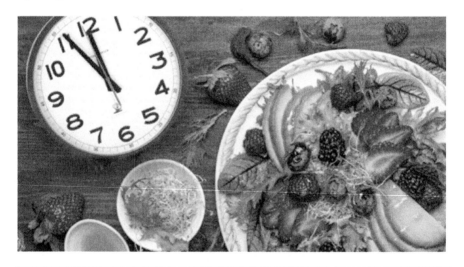

1. 5:2 Fasting

This is one of most widely used IF methods. In reality, the book The FastDiet popularised it and explains all you need to know about it. The plan is to diet regularly for five days (without counting calories) and then consume 500 or 600 calorie intake a day for men and women, respectively, for the remaining two days. The fasting days can be any days you like.

Short fasting periods are thought to keep you compliant; if you get hungry on a quick day, just think of tomorrow when you will "feast" again. "Some people think, 'I can do something for two days, but cutting back on what I consume for seven days is too much,'" Kumar says. For these individuals, a 5:2 approach could be preferable to calorie restriction during the week.

The writers of The FastDiet, though, warn against fasting for days where you're performing a lot of endurance exercise. If you are practising for a cycling or running event (or a high-mileage week), see a sports nutritionist to see if this style of fasting can fit with your training schedule.

2. Time-Restricted Fasting

This type of IF requires you to choose an eating window per day, which should leave you with a 14 to 16 hour fast. (Shemek advises women to fast for no longer than 14 hours a day due to hormonal concerns.) "Fasting encourages autophagy, the body's normal 'cellular housekeeping' process that starts when liver glycogen is exhausted and clears debris and other items that get in the way of mitochondrial health," Shemek says. According to her, doing so can help maximise fat cell metabolism and optimise insulin function.

Set the eating window, for example, from 9 AM to 5 PM to make this work. According to Kumar, this works really well for anyone who has a family who eats an early dinner anyway. And there's the fact that most of the time spent fasting is spent sleeping. (Depending on where you scheduled your window, you still don't have to "skip" any meals.) However, this is based on the ability to remain consistent. Regular times of fasting might not be for you if your life is constantly shifting, or if you want or need the freedom to go out to brunch on occasion, go on a late date night, or go to happy hour.

3. Overnight Fasting

This method is the most basic of the bunch, and it requires fasting for 12 hours a day. For instance, choose to avoid eating after dinner at 7 p.m. and start eating at 7 a.m. the next morning with breakfast. At the 12-hour stage, autophagy also occurs, but the cellular benefits are milder, according to Shemek. This is the bare minimum of fasting hours she advises.

This approach has the advantage of being simple to execute. You really don't have to miss meals; what you're doing is cutting out a bedtime snack (whether you've only eaten one). However, this approach would not fully exploit the benefits of fasting. If you're fasting to lose weight, a narrower fasting window ensures you'll have more food to feed, and does not make you ingest less calories.

4. Eat Stop Eat

In his book Eat Stop Eat; Shocking Truth That Makes Weight Loss Simple Again, author Brad Pilon introduced this technique. His strategy varies from some in that it stresses versatility. Simply stated, he stresses that fasting is nothing more than a temporary abstinence from food. You stick to a resistance conditioning programme and 1 or 2, 24-hour fasts per week. "When your quick is done, I want you to eat responsibly and act as though it never occurred. That is what there is to it. "I don't do much else," he claims on his webpage.

Eating wisely involves returning to a regular eating routine in which you don't binge when you've already fasted, but you still don't neglect yourself or consume less than you require. According to Pilon, the safest method for fat loss is intermittent fasting mixed with routine weight exercise. You will consume a marginally larger number of calories on the other 5 to 6 nonfasting days whether you go on one of two 24-hour fasts throughout the week. He claims that this allows it smoother and more fun to finish the week in a calorie shortage without feeling compelled to go on a strict diet.

5. Whole Day Fasting

You just eat once a day here. According to Shemek, certain people prefer to consume dinner and not eat again before the next day's dinner. That means you'll be fasting for 24 hours. This is not the same as the 5:2 method. Fasting times are usually 24 hours (dinner to dinner / lunch to lunch), while 5:2 needs a 36-hour fast. (For example, you could eat dinner on Sunday, then go on a 500-600 calorie fast on Monday before breaking it with breakfast on Tuesday.)

The benefit is that, if achieved for weight reduction, eating a whole day's worth of calories in one sitting is very difficult (though not impossible). The downside of this strategy is that it's difficult to provide all of the nutrition your body needs with only one meal. Not to mention, sticking to this strategy is difficult. By the time dinner arrives, you may be ravenous, leading you to eating less-than-healthy, calorie-dense foods. Consider this: When you're hungry, broccoli isn't really the first thing that comes to mind. According to Shemek, often people consume too much coffee to satisfy their hunger, which may disrupt their sleep. If you don't eat, you can feel brain fog throughout the day.

6. Fasting on alternate days

Krista Varady, Doctorate, a nutrition professor at university of Illinois in Chicago, popularised this approach. People can fast every other day, with such a fast consisting of 25% of their daily calorie requirements (approximately 500 calories) but nonfasting days being regular eating days. This is a common weight-loss strategy. In reality, Dr. Varady and colleagues observed that alternate-day fasting was successful in helping obese adults lose weight in a limited study reported in Nutrition Journal. By week two, the participants' side effects (such as hunger) had died down, and by week four, they were becoming more satisfied on the diet.

The drawback is that participants claimed they were never really "complete" over the eight weeks of the study, which may render sticking to this plan challenging.

7. Choose Your Day Fasting

It's more like a pick-your-own adventure here. According to Shemek, you can do time-restricted fasting every other day or once a day or twice a week (fast for 16 hours, feed for eight, for example). That means you could have a regular day of eating on Sunday and quit eating by 8 p.m., then start eating again at noon on Monday. It's the equivalent to missing breakfast a couple times a week.

Something to keep in mind: The literature on the impact of missing breakfast is mixed, according to an article reported of the journal Critical Reports in Food Science & Nutrition in December 2015. While several studies suggest that consuming it leads to a lower BMI, there is no clear proof in randomised trials that it causes weight loss. Other studies, such as one reported in the Journal of American College of Cardiology in October 2017, have connected missing breakfast to worse cardiac health.

This is more able to adapt to your lifestyle and goes with the breeze, because you can make things fit even though the routine varies week to week. However, looser methods can result in only minor benefits.

Chapter: 3 Health Benefits of Intermittent Fasting

Intermittent fasting is an eating practice under which you alternate between eating and fasting periods.

Intermittent fasting can be done in a variety of ways, such as the 16/8 or 5:2 techniques. Numerous studies have shown that it can have significant health and cognitive effects.

Here are ten health effects of prolonged fasting that have been scientifically proven.

1. Intermittent fasting changes Cell, Genes, and Hormone Function

When you don't eat for a bit, the body goes through a number of changes.

To render accumulated body fat more available, the body, for example, initiates essential cellular repair processes, changes hormone levels.

Here are some of the physiological modifications that arise during fasting:

- **Insulin levels:** Insulin levels in the blood decrease dramatically, allowing fat to be burned more efficiently.

- **Human growth hormone:** Growth hormone levels in the blood will rise by up to fivefold. Increased levels of this hormone promote fat burning and muscle gain, among other things.

- **Cellular repair:** Significant cellular repair mechanisms, such as the removal of excess content from cells, are induced by the body.

- **Gene expression:** There are advantageous variations in a number of genes and molecules that are linked to survival and disease protection.

These improvements in hormones, gene expression, and cell structure are linked to many of the advantages of intermittent fasting.

Insulin levels decrease, and human growth hormone levels rise as you fast. Your cells also activate critical cellular repair processes and change the expression of genes.

2. Intermittent fasting may help weight loss and belly fat loss

Many people who experiment with intermittent fasting do so in order to reduce weight. In general, extended fasting causes you to consume fewer meals. You can need fewer calories unless you compensate for consuming even more during the other meals.

Intermittent fasting often improves hormone function, which helps weight reduction. Lower insulin levels, raising growth hormone levels, and increasing norepinephrine (noradrenaline) levels all help to break down body fat and make it more useful for energy. As a result, short-term fasting boosts your metabolic rate by 3.6 - 14%, helping you to consume more calories.

Intermittent fasting, in other words, operates on all sides of the calorie equation. It raises the metabolic rate (calories expended), thereby decreasing the quantity of food you consume (decreases calories in).

Intermittent fasting, according to a 2014 study of the scientific literature, will result in weight loss of 3-8 percent over 3-24 weeks. This is a massive amount.

The participants have lost 4-7 percent of their waist circumference, indicating that they lost a lot of belly fat, the disease-causing fat in the abdominal cavity.

Intermittent fasting produced less muscle weakness than prolonged calorie restriction, according to a review report. When it is said and done, extended fasting may be a very effective weight-loss strategy.

3. Intermittent fasting Will Help You Avoid Type 2 Diabetes by Reducing Insulin Resistance

In recent decades, type 2 diabetes has become extremely widespread.

High blood sugar levels in the sense of insulin resistance are the most prominent feature. Something that lowers insulin tolerance and protects against type 2 diabetes should significantly lower blood sugar levels.

Intermittent fasting has been found to have significant benefits for insulin tolerance and to result in a significant decrease in blood sugar levels. Intermittent fasting has been shown to lower fasting blood sugar by 3-6 percent and fasting insulin by 20-31 percent in human trials.

Intermittent fasting often prevented diabetic rats from kidney injury, which is one of the most serious consequences of diabetes.

This means that intermittent fasting could be very beneficial for individuals at risk of having type 2 diabetes.

There might, still, be certain gender differences. During a 22-day intermittent fasting protocol, blood sugar balance in women actually worsened, according to one report.

4. Intermittent Fasting may Lower Inflammation & Oxidative Stress in the Body

Oxidative stress one of the factors that contribute to aging and the development of a lot of chronic diseases. It contains reactive molecules known as free radicals, which react with and destroy other essential molecules such as protein and DNA.

Intermittent fasting has been shown in some trials to improve the body's tolerance to oxidative stress.

In addition, research indicates that intermittent fasting can help tackle inflammation, which is a major cause of a variety of diseases.

5. Intermittent fasting may well be good for your heart

Heart disease is still the leading cause of death worldwide.

Various health indicators (also regarded as "risk factors") have been linked to an elevated or reduced risk of heart failure.

Intermittent fasting has been shown to increase blood pressure, blood triglycerides, total & LDL cholesterol, inflammation markers, and blood sugar levels, among other risk factors.

However, a significant portion of this is focused on animal research. Before any decisions can be developed, further research on the impact on heart health in humans is needed.

6. Intermittent fasting triggers a variety of cellular repair mechanisms

When we fast, our bodies' cells begin a cellular "waste removal" mechanism known as autophagy. Broken and damaged proteins that accumulate within cells over time are broken down and metabolized by the cells.

Increased autophagy has been linked to a reduction in the risk of cancer and Alzheimer's disease.

7. Intermittent fasting can help in cancer prevention

Cancer is a horrific disease that is marked by uncontrollable cell development. Fasting has been found to have a number of metabolic benefits, including a lower incidence of cancer.

Intermittent fasting can help reduce cancer, according to encouraging results from animal trials. Human studies are required.

Fasting minimized multiple side effects of chemotherapy in human cancer patients, according to some evidence.

8. Intermittent fasting is beneficial to your Brain

What is healthy for the body is frequently often good for the brain. Intermittent fasting increases a number of biochemical characteristics that are linked to brain health.

Reduced oxidative stress, inflammation, blood sugar levels, and insulin resistance are all part of this. Intermittent fasting has been shown in some experiments in rats to accelerate the development of new nerve cells, which could improve brain activity.

It often boosts amounts of a brain hormone named (BDNF), which means brain-derived neurotrophic factor, which lack has been linked to depression and other mental illnesses.

Intermittent fasting also defends against brain injury caused by strokes, according to animal reports.

9. Intermittent fasting can assist in the prevention of Alzheimer's disease

The most prevalent neurodegenerative disorder in the world is Alzheimer's disease. Since there is no treatment for Alzheimer's disease, stopping it from developing in the first place is crucial.

Intermittent fasting can postpone the onset of Alzheimer's disease or minimize its intensity, according to a rat report.

A dietary intervention that involved regular short-term fasts was able to substantially enhance Alzheimer's symptoms in 9 out of 10 patients, according to a series of case studies.

Fasting may also guard against some neurodegenerative disorders, such as Parkinson's and Huntington's disease, according to animal research. However, further human research is required.

10. Intermittent fasting will help you live longer by extending your life span

One of the most intriguing applications of intermittent fasting is the potential to prolong life expectancy.

Intermittent fasting increases longevity in rats in the same manner as constant calorie restriction would. The results of some of these experiments were very dramatic. One of them found that rats who fasted every other day lived 83 percent longer than rats who didn't fast.

Intermittent fasting has been very common with the anti-aging crowd, despite the fact that it has yet to be demonstrated in humans. With the effects of intermittent fasting for metabolism and a variety of health indicators, it's easy to see how it might help you live a longer and happier life.

Chapter: 4 Nine Potential Intermittent Fasting Side Effects

People use the word intermittent fasting to explain dietary habits that include regular cycles of fasting where they intake very few or no calories.

If you are thinking of giving intermittent fasting a chance, you are possibly curious if it has any negative effects.

Intermittent fasting is healthy for the majority of people, according to the brief response. Intermittent fasting does, though, have a few minor side effects, according to research. Furthermore, it is not suitable for everybody.

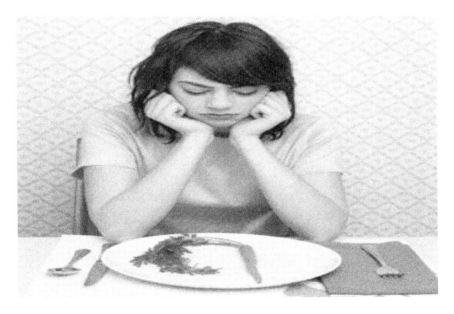

The nine possible side effects of intermittent fasting are addressed in this section.

1. Cravings and Hunger

Hunger is among the most frequent side effects of intermittent fasting, which comes as no surprise. You can feel increased hunger if you limit your calorie consumption or go through large spells without eating.

Any 112 individuals were randomly allocated to an intermittent energy limitation category in a survey. For a year, they ate 400 to 600 calories on two non-consecutive days per week. These individuals reported feeling more hungry than someone that followed a low-calorie diet of constant calorie restriction.

According to studies, hunger is a common symptom people feel within the first few days of a fasting period.

In a 2020 survey, 1,422 participants took part in fasting regimens that lasted 4–21 days. And within the first two days of the regimens, did they feel hunger symptoms.

As a result, hunger symptoms can disappear as your body adjusts to normal fasting periods.

2. Light-headedness and headaches

Intermittent fasting is also associated with headaches. They are most common in the first several days of a fasting protocol.

In a study published in 2020, researchers looked at 18 experiments of people who practiced intermittent fasting. Any researchers of the four trials who reported side effects claimed they had moderate headaches.

Researchers discovered that "fasting headaches" were normally located in the frontal area of the brain, with the discomfort that is mild to moderate in intensity.

Furthermore, those who often suffer from headaches are more prone to suffer from headaches when fasting than others who do not.

Low blood sugar & caffeine withdrawal have been linked to headaches during fasting, according to studies.

3. Digestive Problems

If you do intermittent fasting, you can have digestive problems such as constipation, diarrhea, nausea, and bloating.

The decrease in food consumption that certain intermittent fasting regimens entail can have a detrimental impact on your digestion, resulting in constipation and other unpleasant side effects. Furthermore, dietary modifications connected with intermittent fasting programs may result in bloating and diarrhea.

Constipation may be exacerbated by dehydration, another frequent side effect of intermittent fasting. As a result, it's important to remain well hydrated when fasting intermittently.

Constipation may be avoided while eating nutrient-dense, fiber-rich diets.

4. Irritability as well as other Mood Changes

When people undergo intermittent fasting, they can feel irritability or other mood changes. When your blood sugar is down, you can get irritable.

Hypoglycemia, or low blood sugar, may occur during times of calorie restriction or fasting. Irritability, fear, and low attention are also possible outcomes.

A 2016 analysis of 52 women showed that during an 18-hour fasting cycle, participants were slightly more irritable than during a nonfasting period.

Interestingly, the researchers discovered that, although the women became irritable at the conclusion of the fasting period, they still felt a greater sense of accomplishment, dignity, and self-control than they did at the beginning.

5. Low Energy and Fatigue

Any people who practice different forms of intermittent fasting feel nausea and reduced energy levels, according to studies.

Intermittent fasting can make you feel tired and weak due to low blood sugar. In addition, intermittent fasting can induce sleep disruptions in some people, resulting in fatigue throughout the day.

Intermittent fasting, on the other hand, has been shown in several studies to minimize exhaustion, especially when your body adapts to daily fasting periods.

6. Breath Problems

Bad breath is an unfortunate side effect that certain people experience when they fast intermittently. This is due to a decrease in salivary flow and an increase in acetone in the breath.

Fasting allows the body to burn fat as a source of energy. Since acetone is a by-product of fat synthesis, it rises in your blood and air as you fast.

Dehydration, which is a result of intermittent fasting, may often trigger dry mouth, which may contribute to poor breath.

7. Disturbances of Sleep

According to some studies, sleep disorders, such as the inability to fall or remain asleep, are one of the most frequent side effects of intermittent fasting.

In a 2020 survey, 1,422 participants took part in fasting regimens that lasted 4–21 days. Fasting caused sleep disorders in 15% of the subjects, according to the report. This was mentioned more often than other side effects.

Since the body excretes huge quantities of salt and water by the urine, fatigue can be more normal in the early days of an intermittent fasting regimen. Dehydration & low salt levels will result as a result of this. Some reports, on the other hand, also shown that intermittent fasting has little impact on sleep.

Research published in 2021 looked at 31 obese individuals who fasted on alternating days while still eating a low-carb diet for six months. The research discovered that this routine had little effect on sleep efficiency, length, or the intensity of insomnia.

8. Dehydration

As previously said, the body loses a lot of water and salt in the urine during the first few days of fasting. This is referred to as normal diuresis or fasting natriuresis.

You could get dehydrated if anything occurs to you because you don't recover the fluids and electrolytes you lose by urine.

In addition, people who practice intermittent fasting can fail to drink or drink insufficiently. This is particularly true when you first start an intermittent fasting program.

Drink water during the day and keep an eye on the color of the urine to remain well hydrated. It should ideally be the color of pale lemonade. You could be dehydrated if your urine is dark in color.

9. Malnutrition

Intermittent fasting, if performed incorrectly, will result in malnutrition.

Malnutrition may occur when an individual fast for long periods of time and does not replenish their body with enough nutrients. The same can be said about unplanned, long-term energy restriction diets.

On different forms of intermittent fasting programs, people are usually able to satisfy their calorie and nutritional requirements. However, if you don't properly schedule or execute the fasting diet for a long period of time, or if you intentionally limit calories to an excessive amount, you risk malnutrition and other health problems.

That's why, when fasting intermittently, it's important to eat a well-balanced, healthy diet. Be sure you're not restricting your calorie consumption too far.

A healthcare provider who is familiar with intermittent fasting will assist you in developing a healthy diet that offers the correct number of calories and nutrients for you.

Last but not least

Intermittent fasting has been attributed to a variety of health effects, including reduced heart attack risk factors, weight loss, better blood sugar regulation, and more.

Intermittent fasting is usually thought to be safe, but tests have shown that it can trigger hunger, irritability, constipation, headaches, and bad breath.

In addition, several healthcare providers warn against intermittent fasting. Women who are nursing, chest feeding or breastfeeding, as well as those who have eating disorders, fall under this category.

If you are thinking of attempting intermittent fasting, talk to the doctor first to make sure it's a secure and healthy option for you.

Chapter: 5 Best Foods to Eat on Intermittent Fasting

Please consult a health professional before making any major dietary changes to ensure that it is the right choice for you. Intermittent fasting (IF) is making quite an uproar due to the overcrowding world of dieting, including the phrase "fasting" sounding quite ominous.

A fair amount of research (although with small sample sizes) shows that the diet can help people lose weight and control their blood sugar levels. A reliable source It's no surprise that everybody and their aunt have jumped on the IF bandwagon.

Maybe the attraction stems from the absence of diet restrictions: you can eat what you want, but not exactly when you want. However, it's still necessary to consider what's at stake. Should you be breaking your easy with pints of ice cream & bags of chips? Very likely not. That's why we've compiled a collection of the best things to eat on an IF diet.

Lauren Harris-Pincus, RDN, MS, author of The Protein-Packed Breakfast Club, states, "There are no specifications or limitations on what kind or how much food to consume when practicing intermittent fasting."

However, RDN, Mary Purdy, MS, chair of Dietitians of Integrative & Functional Medicine, counters that " benefits [of IF] are unlikely to follow consistent Big Mac meals."

A well-balanced diet, according to Pincus and Purdy, is the secret to gaining weight, retaining energy levels, and keeping to the diet.

"Anyone trying to reduce weight should eat nutrient-dense foods such as fruits, vegetables, nuts, whole grains, beans, seeds, dairy, and lean proteins," Pincus recommends.

"This guideline will be somewhat similar to the foods I would usually prescribe for better health, high-fiber, unprocessed, entire foods that provide quality and flavor," Purdy says.

To put it another way, if you consume a lot of the foods mentioned below, you won't go hungry when fasting.

1. Water

Well, so this isn't actually a meal, but it's incredibly necessary for surviving IF.

Water is important for the protection of almost all of your body's main organs. Avoiding this as part of the quick will be stupid. Your lungs play a vital role in keeping you safe.

The amount of water that each individual can drink depends on their gender, height, weight, level of exercise, and environment. However, the color of the urine is a strong indicator. For all times, you like it to be pale yellow. Dehydration, which may induce headaches, nausea, and light-headedness, is shown by dark yellow urine. When you combine it with a lack of calories, you have a formula for catastrophe — or, at the very minimum, really dark pee.

If plain water doesn't appeal to you, try adding a splash of lemon juice, several mint leaves, or cucumber slices to it.

The above are some of the reasons why H2O water is the best.

2. Avocado

Eating the highest-calorie fruit when seeking to lose weight can seem counter - intuitive. Avocados, on the other side, can hold you complete through even the most rigorous fasting periods due to its excellent unsaturated fat content.

Unsaturated fats, according to research, help hold the body healthy even though you don't feel hungry. Your body sends out signals that it doesn't need to go into urgent starvation mode because it has enough calories. And if you're starving in the midst of a fasting time, unsaturated fats hold these symptoms are running much longer.

Another research showed that using half an avocado with your lunch will hold you satisfied for up to three hours longer than if you don't consume the green, mushy gem.

3. Seafood and Fish

There's an explanation why the American Dietary Guidelines recommend two or three 4-ounce portions of fish each week. In addition to being high in good fats and proteins, it is also high in vitamin D.

And if you like to feed at short window times, don't you want to get more nutritious bang for your buck while you do?

You will no run out of ways to prepare fish since there are too many options.

4. Cruciferous Veggies

The f-word — fiber — is abundant in foods like brussels sprouts, broccoli, and cauliflower. (We see what you're saying, and no, the f-word doesn't stand for "farts.")

It is important to consume fiber-rich foods at frequent intervals to keep you regular & ensure that your poop factory goes smoothly. Fiber will also help you feel whole, which is useful if you can't feed for another 16 hours. Woof.

Cruciferous vegetables will also help you avoid cancer. Here's where you can learn something about anticancer foods.

5. Potatoes

Repeat after us: White foods aren't all evil.

In the 1990s, the researchers discovered that potatoes are one of the most nutritious foods. In addition, a 2012 study showed that using potatoes in a balanced diet can help weight loss. (Sorry, but potato chips and fries don't count.)

6. Legumes and Beans

On the IF diet, your favorite chili topping might be your best friend.

Food, especially carbohydrates, provides energy for physical exercise. We're not suggesting you go crazy with carbohydrates, so including simple calories like legumes & beans in your diet can't hurt. This will help you stay awake through your fasting period.

Furthermore, ingredients like black beans, chickpeas, peas, and lentils have been proven to help people lose weight, particularly though they aren't on a diet.

7. Probiotics

Can you realize what the gut critters favor? Both consistency and variety are essential. If they are starving, this means they're not comfortable. And if your stomach isn't comfortable, you may notice any unpleasant side effects, such as constipation.

Add probiotic-rich ingredients to the diet, such as kefir, kombucha, and sauerkraut, to combat this unpleasantness.

8. Berries

These smoothie classics are packed with vitamins and minerals. That's not even the most exciting aspect.

People who ate a lot of flavonoids, such as those used in blueberries & strawberries, had lower BMI rises over a 14-year cycle than people who didn't eat berries, according to a 2016 report.

9. Eggs

One big egg has 6.24 grams of protein and takes just minutes to cook. And, particularly when you are eating less, having as much protein as necessary is important for staying full and building muscle.

Men who had an egg breakfast rather than a bagel have been less hungry & ate less during the day, according to a 2010 survey.

To put it another way, if you are looking for something else to do during your quick, why not hard-boil a couple of eggs? And, when the time is perfect, you should consume them.

10.   Nuts

While nuts are higher in calories than many of the other snacks, they do have something that most snacks do not: healthy fats.

Even don't be concerned with calories! According to a 2012 report, a 1-ounce portion of almonds (approximately, 23 nuts) contains 20% fewer calories than the label claims.

Chewing does not fully break down the cell walls of almonds, according to the report, which keeps a part of the nut safe and prevents it from being absorbed by the body through digestion. As a result, eating almonds might not make as much of a difference in your regular calorie intake as you would think.

11. Whole Grain

Dieting and carbohydrate use tend to fall under two distinct categories. This isn't always the case, as you'll be glad to learn. Since whole grains are high in fiber and nutrition, a small amount would keep you satisfied for a long time.

So, get out of your comfort zone and try farro, spelt, bulgur, Kamut, amaranth, sorghum, millet, or freekeh, a whole-grain utopia.

To see who is the fastest, we pit whole-wheat & white pasta against each other.

Chapter: 6 Avoid Foods if you are trying to Burn Belly Fat

The fact is, getting fat around your midsection is totally natural and very common—having reduced body fat and shredded abs are extremely rare. The problem is about the type of fat you have, is subcutaneous fat, which you can pinch with your fingertips, is less dangerous to your wellbeing than visceral fat, which is found deep inside the abdominal cavity. Elevated cholesterol, heart disease and type 2 diabetes and are only a few of the serious health problems that may be caused by visceral fat.

Fortunately, there are measures you may take to reduce certain dangers (which do not involve following fad diets or engaging in derogatory self-talk). Exercise is essential for a long-term healthier lifestyle and weight loss (target for at least thirty minutes of exercise every day, such as walking), but the foods you consume often play a role. We have compiled a list of 12 foods to stop if you are trying to lose belly fat.

1. Potato Chips & French Fries

Potato chips and French fries are not nutritious or filling, but whole potatoes are. They are rich in calories, and it's convenient to consume too much.

Consumption of potato chips and French fries has been related to weight gain in clinical trials. Potato chips, according to one report, can cause weight gain per serving than any other product.

Furthermore, acrylamides, which cause cancer, can be present in cooked, boiled, or fried potatoes. As a result, simple, boiled potatoes are the better option.

2. Cheese

Saturated fat and calories are abundant in cheese. This is not to suggest that all food is off-limits (we do not know what we would do if we could not get our mint chocolate chip ice cream)—healthy alternatives like skim milk still provide nutrition and calcium to the body. Even if you want to trim down your midsection, do as the French do and avoid processed, shredded cheese in favor of limited amounts of additive-free cheeses.

3. Refined Bread

Refined carbs, such as pasta, cannot be reduced in a balanced diet. Inflammation and weight gain are linked to diets high in "dense acellular carbohydrates," according to one report. Consider Ezekiel bread, rye bread, flaxseed bread, oat bread, or whole wheat bread as a better alternative to the morning bagel. You will experience a change in your energy levels during the day, as well as a longer feeling of fullness.

4. Cereal

Breakfast is sometimes referred to as the essential meal of the day, but if you consume several bowls of cereal in the morning, your GI system won't have enough time to absorb the food properly—not to mention that the high sugar content and added white flour would cause weight gain. Instead, go for whole-grain, low-sugar, high-fiber cereals (The high fiber content can make you stay fuller for longer and support the digestive system move). When it comes to which milk to drink with it, Selvakumar suggests low-fat or skim milk for weight reduction or plant-based milk with cereals (oat, almond and soy).

5. Candy Bars

Candy bars are particularly harmful to one's wellbeing. In a little box, they cram a tonne of added sugar, oils, and processed flour.

Candy bars are calorie-dense and nutritionally deficient. An average-sized chocolate-covered candy bar will have 200 to 300 calories, and extra-large bars can have much more. Candy bars, unfortunately, can be found almost everywhere. They're also conveniently put in supermarkets to entice customers to purchase them on impulse.

Eat a slice of fruit or a couple of nuts instead of a cookie if you're hungry.

6. Cookies, Cakes & Pastries

Pastries, biscuits, and desserts are high in toxic additives such as processed flour and artificial sugar. They can also include trans fats, which are very unhealthy and have been related to a variety of diseases.

Pastries, sweets, and cakes are not really filling, and you would most definitely be hunger soon after consuming them. Instead of reaching for a bite of milk chocolate while you want something delicious, aim for a slice of white chocolate.

7. Pizza

Pizza is a common fast-food option. Commercially prepared pizzas, on the other hand, are very unhealthy. They are rich in calories and often have harmful additives, including processed meat and refined flour.

If you just want a slice of pie, make it at home with better ingredients. Home-made pizza sauce is often better, as store-bought sauces may be high in sugar.

Another choice is to seek out a pizza restaurant that specializes in healthy pizzas.

8. High Calories Coffee Drinks

Coffee comprises a number of biologically active compounds, the most common of which is caffeine. These chemicals, at least in the short term, will improve your metabolism & increase fat burning. However, the disadvantages of adding toxic additives such as artificial milk and sugar overshadow the benefits.

Coffee drinks with a lot of calories are no safer than soda. They're high in empty calories and can easily replace a meal.

If you are looking to lose weight, stick to plain, black coffee. It's also good to add a little cream or milk. Only stay away from sugar, calorie-dense creamers, and other unhealthy ingredients.

9. Soft Drink

Artificial sugars & high-fructose corn syrup are used to sweeten soda, all of which will raise intra-abdominal fat and have excess calories: "Sodas can be stopped entirely to minimize abdominal fat and bloating," Selvakumar advises. "Any remaining sugar would be transformed to fat and ultimately deposited in adipose tissue."

Even if you believe you're selecting the "healthier" choice, the chemically sweet flavor of diet soda stimulates the body to release insulin, which leads to elevated blood sugar and a greater waist circumference.

Bottom line: Stay away from sugary beverages.

10.   Added Sugar with Fruit Juice

Many store-bought fruit drinks, including soda, are loaded with sugars, sweeteners, and even high-fructose corn syrup. The same can be said for smoothies purchased from a supermarket. According to Selvakumar, adipose tissue (where excess sugar is transferred to fat) has an infinite holding space, making it impossible to maintain a flat stomach when you drink sugary fruit juice. Start producing your own juices at home instead of going to the store. Though you will have to tidy up a little bit, you will see a change in the freshness & your waistline will prosper.

11. Alcoholic Beverages (Especially Beer)

Alcohol has around seven calories a gram, which is more than carbohydrates and protein. The proof for the connection between alcohol and weight gain, on the other hand, isn't conclusive.

Drinking small amounts of alcohol seems to be safe and has also been attributed to weight loss. On the other hand, heavy drinking has been linked to gaining weight.

It's also important to consider the kind of alcohol you're drinking. Although beer can make you add weight, consuming wine in moderation can potentially help you lose weight.

12. Ice Cream

Ice cream is very tasty, but it is still very unhealthy. It's rich in calories, and the majority of varieties are high in sugar. A tiny serving of ice cream is good once in a while, but the trouble is that it's way too convenient to eat a large quantity in one sitting.

Make your own ice cream with less sugar and more nutritious ingredients like full-fat yogurt and berries. Additionally, feed yourself a tiny slice and set the ice cream away, so you do not overeat.

Bottom Line

Highly refined junk foods are the worse foods for weight reduction. Added sugar, processed wheat, and/or added fats are common ingredients in these foods.

Read the mark if you're not positive if a meal is safe or not. However, be careful of sugars many labels and health statements that could be false.

Keep in mind the serving sizes as well. Nuts, dried fruit, and cheese, for example, are rich in calories, and it's convenient to consume so many of them.

You should also practice mindful feeding, which involves paying careful attention to each slice, chewing carefully, and keeping track of your hunger. This technique will assist you in controlling your nutritional consumption.

Chapter: 7 MYTHS About Intermittent Fasting

When it comes to misconceptions about intermittent fasting, separate truth from myth; it is important to have the correct information whether you are contemplating or practicing intermittent fasting.

You will be more able to fast correctly if you have the evidence. And if you fast correctly, you will be more likely to see the weight loss, consistent energy, and decreased cravings that have to make intermittent fasting so successful.

There is a lot of misinformation around here, unfortunately. You have already read stuff like: Fasting causes the metabolism to slow down... In short, you can avoid drinking water... Alternatively, fasting causes the muscles to shrivel.

Fasting theories, on the other hand, are not based on science. Rather, they are built on rumor, conjecture, and even a misplaced faith in conventional wisdom.

The major intermittent fasting theories will be debunked today. What is the reason for this? That you will make more wise decisions around intermittent fasting as a health-improvement strategy.

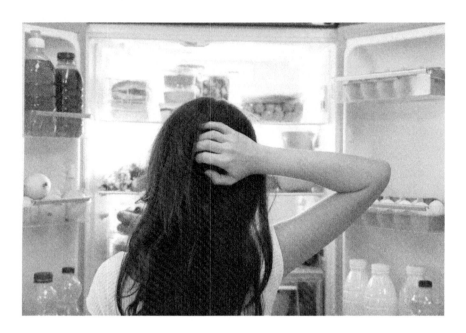

MYTHS about Intermittent Fasting

Now that you know what intermittent fasting is and isn't, it's time to find out what it isn't. Let's debunk those misconceptions of fasting, shall we?

MYTH 1: Fasting Decline Your Metabolism

Some people believe that fasting causes the resting metabolic rate to decrease (To put it another way, fasting causes you to burn few calories at rest). The fear is that if you resume regular eating habits, you'll add weight like such a three-toed sloth.

This is what occurs on calorie-restricted diets, which enable you to consume 50 - 85 % of the calories the body needs on a regular basis for a long time. Your body adjusts to the lower energy consumption and will do so for years.

You have probably seen calorie control in effect on The Biggest Loser. While the contestants lose weight, they nearly always regain it. They never discuss that part of the program, which is inconvenient for viewers.

Is intermittent fasting the same as regular fasting? That does not seem to be the case. Non-obese individuals who exercised alternate-day fasting retained a regular metabolic rate for the majority of 3 weeks, even while burning more fat, according to a 2005 study reported in the American Journal of Clinical Nutrition.

MYTH 2: Do Not Drink Water

Some religious fasts, such as Ramadan fasting, limit all water and food. Unrelated to this, a host of reports have emerged claiming that no-water fasts are beneficial to one's fitness.

Due to the diuretic impact of fasting, restricting water can contribute to serious dehydration. That's why, when supervising clients on surgical fasts, doctors pay particular attention to fluid consumption. Electrolytes, including sodium and potassium, which are also energetically peed out during fasting, are often monitored by doctors.

What's the takeaway? During a fast, drink plenty of water and take potassium and sodium supplements if the fast lasts more than 13 or 14 hours.

MYTH 3: You Can Not Gain Muscle, While Fasting

Fasting would not seem to be the only way to gain muscle strength. Don't you have to pound protein drinks, after all?

Protein is essential, but it is not needed all of the time. In one 2019 report, for Example, active women who fasted 16/8 acquired the same amount of strength and muscle as women who ate on a more traditional schedule.

Here's the deal: In moments of shortage, the body functions overtime to conserve muscle. When you fast, your body fat (rather than muscle) is used to meet your energy needs.

Consider this: if our ancestors burnt through muscle for a long, they would have been unable to hunt.

MYTH 4: Fasting Makes You Overindulgence

You will be hungry after a fast. Many people believe that this hunger would lead to overeating.

The proof, on the other hand, disproves this concern. Ad libitum feeding refers to the process of allowing participants to consume as much as they like during a fasting study. They feed to their hearts' content and still lose weight.

In reality, most intermittent fasting protocols would cause you to consume less rather than more. As a result of the moderate calorie limit, you'll lose weight gradually without slowing down your metabolism.

MYTH 5: It is for Everyone

At the moment, intermittent fasting is quite common. In certain ways, it is marketed as being useful to all, all of the time.

While fasting is generally safe and healthy for the majority of citizens, some groups should avoid it. The below are some of these groups:

- Kids

- Pregnant & nursing mothers

- People who are underweight

The above groups require more food, not less. Fasting's possible gains are outweighed by the chance of nutritional deficiency.

Those with elevated blood sugar should exercise vigilance as well. Fasting may be beneficial for this group, but medical supervision is needed to avoid extremely low blood sugar (hypoglycemia).

MYTH 6: Fasting Depletes the Energy

Food is a source of energy. Would your energy levels plummet if you don't have them?

Yes, ultimately. When you fast intermittently, though, the cells switch to a certain pool of energy: body fat. There's enough of it to go around.

That's right. Even a thin individual (For Example, 150 pounds with 10% body fat) has significant fat reserves to meet energy requirements when fasting. Fifteen pounds of fat equals over sixty-thousand (60,000) calories of energy if you do the calculations.

In reality, many people claim that exercising when fasted gives them more energy. After a big meal, blood is drawn away from tissues and into digestive organs, which makes sense.

MYTH 7: You Can Not Focus While Fasting

Consider the last period you were really hungry. It wasn't likely your most zen moment.

You do not feel this "hangry" condition if you observe intermittent fasting on a daily basis. Your hunger hormones can regulate until your cells have adapted to utilizing body fat for energy.

Ketones are small molecules that provide pure, usable energy to your brain as your burn body fat. It has been shown that promoting ketosis increases concentration, interest, and concentration in older adults.

Bottom Line

It's incredible what this easy and compact eating system will do for the body, brain, and health.

If you move over the common myths of intermittent fasting, you'll notice that many people do more when fasting.

Chapter: 8 Tips for a Successful Intermittent Fasting

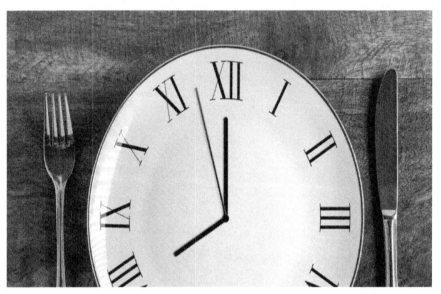

Have you heard of the new eating trend, extended fasting? There's an explanation that so many celebrities do it, and so many others have succeeded in it. This diet isn't even a diet at all; when followed correctly, it can become a routine. Don't be fooled by out-of-date diets like missing meals; we all know they don't work. Intermittent fasting does not entail skipping meals, counting calories, or restricting what you consume (thank goodness!), but only that you want to eat at a certain period of time while fasting during others. It's important to realize that this isn't about deprivation but rather about splitting the calories in a new way.

Intermittent fasting will help you lose weight while still lowering your blood pressure, improving glucose levels, and even slowing down the aging process (yes, this is a thing). When we eat, our insulin levels rise, which converts to accumulated sugar in the liver and causes fat to develop. When we fast, our insulin levels drop, and we burn off the sugar we've stored. To put it another way, if you are always eating, the body will be using the food as energy, which ensures you would never burn the fat you have saved.

Diets can be difficult to follow, take time out from your life, restrict you, and be rather costly. Fasting, on the other hand, lets you simplify your life and is completely healthy. It saves you time by requiring you to cook fewer meals, and it is accessible to you at any time and from any place. There are several good reasons to begin this diet and make it a routine. Of course, before making any big lifestyle changes, you can consult with your doctor! When you're ready to give intermittent fasting a shot, here are ten tips to get you started.

1. Choose the Best Fasting Duration for You

Since the intermittent fast is really adaptable, you must select a style that would work for you. It can be followed in a variety of ways. You have the choice of using the 16:8 or 20:4 scale. The 16:8 method entails fasting for 16 hours a day (a large portion of which would be spent sleeping), followed by an 8-hour window for eating. A 20-hour fast is supplemented by a 4-hour feeding window in the 20:4 cycle. Both of these strategies give you the freedom to start and end them whenever you choose. You might, for example, break the fast at 12 p.m. and eat before 8 p.m. If breakfast is more valuable to you and you have the stamina to avoid evening snacking, a 10 a.m. to 6 p.m. window could be more suitable.

You may also decide on a longer fasting time. This can include the 5:2 diet, which entails eating five days a week and fasting for two days. This diet is so adaptable that you can pick whatever appeals to you or is more realistic for you while also getting the same results.

2. Gradually Start

It is advised to ease into a new diet or lifestyle, such as intermittent fasting. This will assist the body in adapting to a more seamless change. If fasting from your usual breakfast period until 12 p.m. does not work for you, consider increasing it by one hour the first day and two hours the next day till you can go until lunchtime without eating.

Some people will jump straight into something different and push past the hard moments and cravings, but if you're not one of them, start slowly if you want to see results.

3. Ride Out Hunger Waves

Hunger isn't constant; it falls in waves. Try battling out a hunger wave the next time that feels too much to handle. Contrary to popular wisdom, if you get starving, it won't keep heating up until you feel like you're about to explode; it will finally subside, and all you have to do now is get through it.

When hunger hits, it's essential to stay hydrated. Your body could be displaying signs of hunger as a result of dehydration when all you need is some water.

4. Drink a lot of water

As previously said, it is important to consume lots of water when fasting. This not only keeps you hydrated but also makes your stomach feel whole. You are free to consume as much water as you want.

Drinking tea or coffee (but just black; cream and sugar will interrupt your fast) will also help to satisfy any cravings you might have during your fasting period.

5. Don't Binge

When fasting, this is very important. Make an effort to avoid breaking the fast by overeating. When breaking your fast, it can be difficult not to reach for the greatest meal you can find, particularly at the beginning. If you do, you risk eating too quickly, too frequently, and making bad food decisions, all of which can make the body dislike you in the long run.

When it comes to breaking the fast, the easiest way to do is schedule out healthier meals to consume and eat steadily. Begin with a light lunch, and if you get hungry again quickly, try a different snack.

6. Consume Nutritious Foods

This might sound obvious, but make sure you're filling your body with nutritious foods in between fasting times. According to several research, eating a low-carb diet during intermittent fasting will make you feel less hungry.

Not to mention that consuming nutritious foods helps the body feel healthy and gives your mind the energy it needs to think clearly. We've all had the experience of eating a fast-food meal that, while satisfying, leaves you with a feeling of brain fog and makes your body feel heavy and unmotivated for the rest of the day.

7. Keep Yourself Busy

Keeping busy is one of the most effective ways to relieve yourself from what might seem to be hunger. How much of you, like me, notice yourself consuming unnecessarily while bored? This is when you have plenty to take your mind, so you say, "Oh, I'm hungry," though you aren't.

To keep yourself busy, consider taking up a new hobby. Reading books, listening to a podcast, or cleaning the house will all help. Much better, get that booty moving and do a workout to hold yourself busy. Nothing beats adding at least 30 minutes of exercise into your day to promote a healthier lifestyle, not to mention the fact that it can keep you away from calories and helping you feel amazing. If you can't help worrying about food at work, rethink your assignment. Perhaps you ought to take a five-minute mental break to switch tasks; the important thing is to keep busy so that feelings about food don't stick in your mind and put you off track.

8. Journal

This is a fantastic and vital tip, journal! From the start, keep track of everything. If you're a computer geek, use your tablet, but if you're more of a traditionalist like me, keep track in a journal.

Keeping track of your everyday food consumption during non-fasting hours is a smart thing, as is keeping track of your moods, both good and negative, in the process. This way, you'll be able to see how far you've come. It could have been your body getting used to the fresh fasting you've been trying, or it could have been the giant bun you had for lunch that made you furious Monday afternoon. If you don't chart your weight loss or healthier lifestyle journey, it's difficult to know if there are any changes. Take a lot of photographs in addition to monitoring the moods and nutritional consumption. Seeing is the simplest way to believe. Take before and after pictures because you have plenty to look back on and see if you've made some improvement.

9. Get Rid of the Negative People

It's important to tell the right people whether you're following a fresh diet or something that you're particularly curious about. Whether you have a couple of bad people in your life or you know someone has negative feelings, don't bring them out on your new adventure.

When beginning a new diet or lifestyle, it is important to have the correct support system. To help you succeed, you'll need others to assist you, inspire you, and support your new path.

10. Allow a Month

The most key point to remember before beginning every new routine or activity is to allow it time. The proverb "Rome wasn't built in a day" has a lot of meaning. You can't hope to lose a lot of weight by doing extended fasting for a few days.

It takes time for your body to adapt, and it takes time for your mind to become a habit. If you're planning to pursue intermittent fasting, offer it at least a month before determining if it's right for you.

Chapter: 9 Mistakes of Intermittent Fasting

1. Getting started quickly with intermittent fasting

One of the greatest blunders you can make is to start too quickly. You will set yourself up for failure if you dive into IF without first easing into it. It may be difficult to transition from consuming three large meals or six small meals a day to feeding within a four-hour timeframe, for example.

Instead, eventually, introduce fasting. If you choose to use the 16/8 method, gradually increase the period between meals so you can function easily in a 12-hour window. Then, to bring the window down to 8 hours, apply a few minutes per day before you get there.

2. Choosing the Wrong Plan

You have shopped for whole foods like fish, vegetables, chicken, fruits, nutritious sides like legumes and quinoa, and you are excited to pursue Intermittent Fasting for weight loss. The issue is that you haven't selected the IF strategy that will ensure your performance. If you go to the gym six days a week, absolutely fasting on two of those days might not be the best option for you.

Rather than jumping into a strategy without worrying about it, examine your lifestyle and choose the plan that better fits your routine and behaviors.

3. Eating too Much

The shorter time left to consume requires eating fewer calories, which is one of the reasons why people want to pursue Intermittent Fasting. Some participants, on the other hand, will consume their daily number of calories during the fasting window. It's possible that you won't lose weight as a result of this.

Don't consume the daily calorie intake of 2000 calories in the slot. Instead, target for a caloric intake of 1200-1500 calories during the time you're breaking the quick. If you fast for 4, 6, or 8 hours, the number of meals you eat can be determined by the duration of the fasting window. If you find yourself in a state of hunger and need to feed, rethink the diet you want to pursue, or take a day off the IF to refocus and get back on track.

4. Eating Wrong Food

Overeating goes hand and hand with the Intermittent Fasting blunder of choosing the wrong foods. You would not feel good if you have a fasting time of 6 hours and filled it with refined, salty, or sugary foods.

The mainstay of your diet becomes lean meats, good fats, almonds, unrefined grains, legumes, wholesome vegetables and fruits. In addition, while you're not fasting, keep some healthy food ideas in mind:

- Rather than eating at a cafe, prepare and eat at home.

- Read diet labels and learn about additives, including high fructose corn syrup & refined palm oil that aren't allowed.

- Keep an eye out for hidden sugars and limit sodium consumption.

- Instead of refined ingredients, prepare whole foods.

- Fiber, balanced fats and carbohydrates, and lean proteins can all be present on your plate.

5. Restricting Calories

And, there is such a phenomenon as calorie restriction that is excessive. It's not safe to eat fewer than 1200 calories during your fasting window. Not just that, but it has the potential to slow down your metabolic rate. If you delay your metabolism so long, you'll start losing muscle mass instead of gaining it.

To stop making this mistake, plan your meals for the whole week ahead of the weekend. This means you'll already have well-balanced, nutritious meals on hand. When it's time to eat, you can choose from a variety of good, tasty, and calorie-balanced options.

6. Unknowingly Breaking Intermittent Fasting

It's essential to be mindful of hidden quick breakers. Did you realize that even the flavor of sugar makes the brain release insulin? This triggers the release of insulin, essentially breaking the fast. Here are some unexpected foods, supplements, and items that can stop a quick and trigger an insulin response:

- Supplements containing maltodextrin and pectin, as well as other additives

- Sugar and fat are used in supplements such as gummy bear vitamins.

- Using mouthwash and toothpaste containing xylitol as a sweetener

- Sugar can be used in the wrapping of pain relievers like Advil.

Breaking the fast is a common Intermittent Fasting error. When you're not eating, clean your teeth with a baking soda and water mixture, and scan the labels closely before consuming vitamins and supplements.

7. Not Drinking Enough

Suppose necessitates that you stay hydrated. Keep in mind that the body isn't absorbing the water that will normally be absorbed with food. As a result, if you're not patient, side effects might throw you off. If you cause yourself to become dehydrated, you can experience muscle cramps, headaches and extreme hunger.

Include the following in the day to prevent this error to avoid unpleasant signs, including cramping and headaches:

- Water

- 1-2 tbsp apple cider vinegar, with water (this might also help you eat less)

- A cup of black coffee

- Green tea, black tea, herbal tea, or oolong tea

8. Not Exercising

Some people believe they can't exercise during an IF time, when in fact, it's the perfect situation. Exercising makes you burn fat that has been stored in your body. Additionally, when you exercise, the Human Growth Hormone levels increase, assisting in muscle growth. There are, though, certain guidelines to obey in order to get the most out of the workouts.

Keep the following points in mind to get the best possible results from your efforts:

- Time your workouts to coincide with meal times, and then eat healthy carbs and proteins within 30 minutes of finishing your workout.

- If the exercise is painful, make sure you eat beforehand to replenish your glycogen stores.

- Base the workout on the fasting method; if you're fasting for 24 hours, don't do something strenuous that day. Stay hydrated during the quick, particularly throughout the workout.

- Pay attention to your body's signals; if you start to feel weak or light-headed, take a break or stop working out.

9. Too Harsh on Yourself

Failure is not described by a single blunder. You will have days where an IF diet is especially difficult, and you don't think you'll be able to keep up. It's perfectly acceptable to take a break if necessary. Set aside a day to refocus. Stick to the balanced food plan, but indulge in surprises like an amazing protein smoothie or a plate of healthy broccoli and beef the next day.

Don't fall into the trap of having Intermittent Fasting take over your whole life. Consider it a part of your good routine; just don't forget to take care of yourself in other ways. Enjoy a good read, get some exercise, spend more time with your family, and live as healthily as possible. It's just a function of being the strongest version of yourself.

Chapter: 10 Intermittent Fasting and Keto

When you combine two popular approaches, you'll get better outcomes. Is it, therefore, feasible to continue — and adhere to — this combined strategy?

Cutting carbohydrates and replacing them with fat is gaining popularity. However, if you've had success losing weight with this popular approach, known as the ketogenic diet (or keto for short), you may be considering mixing keto with intermittent fasting to break through a plateau or better your outcomes. Is this something you can take a chance on?

The short response is yes, but you should be aware that this technique hasn't been thoroughly researched or shown to function for weight loss. According to experts, it might make sense, but due to a lack of testing, you can think twice before pursuing this eating strategy.

According to Lori Shemek, Ph.D., a wellness and weight loss specialist in Dallas and author of How to Fight FATflammation, combining the two diets gained attention after intermittent fasting specialist Jason Fung, MD, author of The Obesity Code, suggested utilizing keto as a basis for fasting. According to Dr. Shemek, celebrities such as Halle Berry are reported to follow the diet.

Let's take a look at what each diet entails.

10.1 Basics of Ketogenic Diet

According to previous studies, scientists developed the keto diet in the 1920s to better control seizures in children with epilepsy. According to Epilepsy Foundation, this variant, known as the "traditional" keto diet or the "long-chain triglyceride diet," allows for consuming 3 to 4 gram (g) of fat for every 1 gram of carbs and protein.

The variation of keto that many people are using for weight reduction today is a moderate-protein, high-fat and very-low-carb diet. Fat comprises around 80% of your daily calories, and you can target 20 to 50 grams of carbs (carbs minus fiber) per day, depending on your needs.

Many carbohydrates, like nutritious items including fiber-rich whole grains and certain vegetables, are avoided on the keto diet in favour of fats like olive oil, grass-fed beef, avocado and even bacon on occasion.

The aim of this diet plan is to change your body from burning glucose (or carbs) for energy to burning fat for energy. Ketosis, or being keto-adapted, is the term for this condition.

In the near term, the keto diet will certainly result in rapid weight loss. However, opponents point out that there is a shortage of long-term evidence (more than 2 years) on individuals who use keto for weight reduction.

Many of the arguments that keto can manage health problems other than epilepsy — like elevated blood pressure, diabetes, cancer, polycystic ovary syndrome (PCOS) & neurological disorders, including Alzheimer's disease.

10.2 Intermittent Fasting with Keto

Keto or IF can help you lose weight in the short term, but all diets are very rigid, so they aren't for everybody.

So, what if you combined them? Is it possible that two is greater than one?

First, some scholars believe that combining the two methods makes sense. The keto diet raises ketones levels in the body, and ketones are often increased during fasting periods. "When you're in caloric ketosis, the brain uses less glucose for energy. As a result, after a few weeks of consuming low-carb or ketogenic, the change into a fasted (ketogenic) condition during the day becomes seamless," says Dominic D'Agostino, Ph.D., associate professor at University of South Florida in Tampa & creator of KetoNutrition.org.

At the Cleveland Clinic's Functional Ketogenics Program, physicians advise patients about this technique. According to Logan Kwasnicka, a licensed physician assistant at Cleveland Clinic in Ohio, "adding intermittent fasting will take it to the next level." Since people consume fewer calories while doing IF, the next step could be breaking through a weight loss plateau, it may also be a gradual progression from a keto diet to those who are not disturbed by their eating window narrowing and feel satiated eating too much fat (ketosis can also decrease appetite).

10.3 Who Could Try a Keto Intermittent Fasting Diet?

Anyone who's been on keto for more than 2 weeks and wants to add IF will do so with the permission of their healthcare staff. However, the keto diet has become common with people with prediabetes or diabetes, despite the fact that "asking such patients not to feed for an extended period of time may be dangerous," according to Kwasnicka. It's doubtful that you'll be a successful match for this combined diet schedule whether you have kidney disease, a background of eating disorders, are under active cancer treatment, or are pregnant or breastfeeding. Individual diets (keto and IF) might not be appropriate for these people. Consult with the medical staff.

You still don't need to add more IF, if you're still on the keto diet and comfortable about how you're eating, she says.

10.4 Best Way to Start Keto Intermittent Fasting Diet

At the Cleveland Clinic, doctors caution against starting keto and intermittent fasting at the same time. "Changing from glucose to ketones as a big shock to the brain, and applying IF is a major change," Kwasnicka notes. As a result, people will begin with keto. They may think It after a couple of weeks or months on a diet.

It's also essential to choose the correct time. Kwasnicka recommends a 12 to 16 hour easy for their patients. Not eating for 12 hours a day (say, from 7 pm to 7 am) is a natural activity for many people and does not necessitate skipping meals.

To begin, Shemek recommends delaying breakfast (beginning with an hour and gradually increasing the time) to get your body used to go long periods without eating. Reintroduce breakfast earlier in the day and prolong your nighttime fasting period until you've adjusted to the current eating schedule, as eating breakfast not only improves memory but also metabolism and insulin sensitivity, according to a report reported in the month of August year 2018 in the American Journal of Physiology-Endocrinology Metabolism. She advises doing keto-IF for no longer than six months before switching to a more traditional low-carb diet.

10.5 Steps to Getting Started with Keto Intermittent Fasting

1) Get Used to Intermittent Fasting

The easiest way to get started with keto intermittent fasting is to take things slowly at first.

- Start with a couple of days of 16/8 intermittent fasting and without making any adjustments to your diet if you're new to fasting.

- If you have fasted before and are comfortable doing so, you should skip this phase and move straight to make dietary adjustments.

Our 21-Day Keto Fasting Action Plan recommends steadily of the eating window to help your body adjust to intermittent fasting. On the very first day, you begin with 12-hour fast & eventually increase it to 16 hours.

What is the best way to choose your keto fasting?

For many people, missing breakfast is the most convenient choice, although some people choose to miss dinner instead. A few possible 16/8 keto intermittent fasting scenarios include:

1. Start fasting around 4 p.m. if you begin eating at 8 a.m.

2. Start fasting around 8 p.m., if you begin eating at 12 p.m.

3. If you begin eating at 2 p.m., avoid eating & begin fasting at 10 p.m.

2) Explain the Keto Diet: What Do You Eat?

Do you have confidence in your ability to adhere to your intermittent fasting plan? This is fantastic. The ketogenic diet would be the next phase in adjusting your nutrition.

Decide if you'll adhere to a 5/70/25 large nutritional breakdown or calculate net carbs only while following the keto diet (read more here).

The foods that are suggested for the keto IF diet are mentioned below.

Foods that are Keto Intermittent Fasting Friendly

All below foods with a minimal or low crab ratio, such as:

- Salmon, mackerel, and sardines are high-fat seafood.

- Meat that has not been processed, such as beef, pork, lamb, and poultry

- Eggs

- Oils

- Full-fat dairy products & butter

- Vegetables that are green and leafy

- Pecan, Brazil, and Macadamia Nuts

- Berries are a kind of berry that is (in moderation).

Foods to avoid on the Keto Intermittent Fast

All foods of 10 grams or more of carbs per 100 grams should be avoided, including:

- Wheat, barley, corn, rye, buckwheat quinoa, and bulgur are examples of grains and starches.

- Pasta, cereal, bread, pastries, oatmeal, muesli, and pizza are also grain items.

- Beans, lentils, chickpeas and peas are examples of legumes.

- Potatoes, parsnips, sweet potatoes, and yams are also rooted vegetables.

- The majority of fruits.

- Sweetened beverages, such as sauces, beer, and juice, include sugar.

To keep under the appropriate macro guidelines, you should also restrict your consumption of some fruits, dairy products, nuts, and seeds.

3) How Can You Work Out Your Net Carbs?

You may have learned that not all carbs are created equal. It's important to remember that net carbs, not total carbs, are important in the keto diet.

You may be wondering what net carbs are. The cumulative number of carbs consumed by your body is known as net carbs. Fiber, which is used in most whole foods and flows straight through the intestine, is deducted while calculating net carbs.

Check the nutritious value of unpackaged & unprocessed foods like nuts, fruits, vegetables, meat, and others online.

Net carbs are measured by subtracting fiber from overall carbs on processed goods with a Nutritional Facts mark.

Nutrition Facts
8 servings per container
Serving size   **2/3 cup (55g)**

Amount per serving
Calories   230

	% Daily Value*
Total Fat 8g	10%
Saturated Fat 1g	5%
Trans Fat 0g	
Cholesterol 0mg	0%
Sodium 160mg	7%
Total Carbohydrate 37g	13%
Dietary Fiber 4g	14%
Total Sugars 12g	
Includes 10g Added Sugars	20%
Protein 3g	
Vitamin D 2mcg	10%
Calcium 260mg	20%
Iron 8mg	45%
Potassium 235mg	6%

* The % Daily Value (DV) tells you how much a nutrient in a serving of food contributes to a daily diet. 2,000 calories a day is used for general nutrition advice.

NET CARBOHYDRATE =
TOTAL CARBOHYDRATE – DIETARY FIBER

Net carbs = Total carbs – Fiber

4) How to Reach Ketosis?

- When you eat a low-carb diet, the body can naturally enter a state of ketosis. The amount of glucose emitted decreases as carb consumption decreases. As a result, the body switches from using glucose as an energy source to consuming stored fat.

- It's just as important to eat more fat as it is to eat fewer carbs. Food fat promotes ketone production while still keeping you energized.

- Getting enough protein in your diet Protein does not, though, become the key component of your diet since it can allow the body to enter gluconeogenesis. When the body absorbs glucose from protein, gluconeogenesis kicks you out of ketosis.

Since beginning a keto intermittent fasting diet, you can achieve ketosis within 12 hours to 7 days.

5) Typical Day on Keto Intermittent Faster

Do you ever wonder what a normal day of eating on a keto intermittent fasting plan looks like?

The explanation below is for the 16/8 fasting process; however, you may normally change it to suit your needs.

- 8 AM: A cup of black tea or coffee

- 12 PM (Noon): Pan-fried chicken breast with avocado oil, eaten with buttery sauteed spinach

- 3 PM: Keto strawberry chia seed & flax seed pudding

- 8 PM: Dill-infused baked salmon with buttery parmesan, asparagus, and sliced almonds.

6) How Do You Realize If You're In Ketosis?

Since our bodies are all different, one of us can achieve ketosis sooner than the other. You should use one of the three methods below to decide whether you've achieved ketosis and what your ketone levels are:

- Using keto strips to analyze urine

- Via a blood test

- Using ketone breath analyzers, a quick breath is taken.

Though donating blood every day is too time-consuming and costly, urine strips & breath analyzers are more effective at-home alternatives.

We favor the accuracy and convenience of breath ketone monitors over the other two choices. They're convenient to use on the go (without any need to run to the toilet while you're at college and/or take test kits with you), and they let you test the consistency of your diet as many times as you like during the day.

7) Who Shouldn't Do Keto Intermittent Fasting?

Before you pursue keto intermittent fasting, there's one last thing to think about: if it's a safe solution for you.

Although Keto Intermittent Fasting is generally safe for most healthy people, there are some people who should avoid it, particularly:

- If you have asthma.

- If you take blood pressure or heart attack drugs.

- If you have a background of disordered eating.

- If you are pregnant or breastfeeding.

- When you are under the age of 18

- You are having trouble sleeping.

It goes without mentioning that if you have a medical problem or are confused, you can still contact your doctor to determine if Keto Intermittent Fasting is appropriate for you and for how long.

Another factor to keep in mind is that a low-carb diet cannot be followed for an extended period of time. It is a perfect way to lose weight quickly and boost your fitness, but it is not a diet that can be followed indefinitely.

10.6 Health Benefits of Keto Intermittent Fasting Diet's

While there is little evidence on the health benefits of combining keto and intermittent fasting, it is apparent that ketone levels rise as the two diets are mixed. According to Dr. D'Agostino, this might help you lose weight faster. Still, when everybody reacts differently, he notes, this might not be accurate for everyone.

Shemek recommends keto or a combination of IF and keto to all of her clients. "The majority of my clients are prediabetic and overweight. They will quickly stick to an IF and keto diet until they see and realize what eating this way does for them, like controlling their blood sugar levels. "Their commitment is strengthened by the effectiveness of the combined approach," she says.

Instead of weight reduction, one surprising aspect that low-carb IF diets are being researched is for cognitive wellbeing. According to Richard Isaacson, MD, director of the Alzheimer's Prevention Clinic at Weill Cornell Medicine & New York-Presbyterian Hospital in New York City, doing a low-carb, time-restricted IF may help "calm down insulin pathways and enable the brain to benefit from clean-burning [ketone] fuel," which could be useful for people with Alzheimer's disease.

In reality, four or five days a week, Dr. Isaacson does an 8-hour eat, 16-hour fast. According to him, this technique can even help reduce fat accumulation around the waist. He claims that a larger abdomen "could" indicate a smaller memory core in the brain. Furthermore, according to a study reported in the British Journal of Radiology in January 2012, having more visceral (belly) fat is linked to a greater incidence of chronic diseases such as cardiac failure and type 2 diabetes.

10.7 Health Risks of Doing Keto & Intermittent Fasting Together

"People with epilepsy problems (what keto was designed to treat) have been on the keto diet for decades and show exceptional health," D'Agostino says of the long-term complications. However, as in any diet, it all relies on the foods you consume. A keto diet high in bacon and butter is not the same as one high in avocado & olive oil, and a poorly planned keto diet will result in nutritional deficiencies. That IF will force you to dramatically reduce your calorie intake, you may lose much more weight / lean mass (muscle) if you go too far. He advises eating 1 g of protein per kilogram of body weight per day to preserve muscle mass.

Bottom Line

The keto diet is a high-fat diet; low-carb and intermittent fasting limits the period of time you consume. There isn't enough research on either diet alone, let alone this mixed strategy because you don't know what you're getting yourself into whether you pursue them separately or together.

If you plan to try the diets, keep in mind that they are highly restrictive, so sticking to the low carb count and limited eating window can be challenging. (Even children who adopt the ketogenic diet to better manage their seizures struggle to stick to it!)

Consult the healthcare staff before agreeing to combine keto with intermittent fasting. Your doctor will help you determine out how this combination eating plan is right for you, and then they will change the medications you're on to help you succeed in the best way possible.

Chapter: 11 Exercise During Intermittent Fasting

You will learn about anyone performing intermittent fasting (IF) and continuing their exercise routine on every social media plan or online fitness and health publication.

While the IF craze seems to be receiving a lot of attention, this kind of lifestyle isn't unique. There's a lot of studies and anecdotal evidence about how to make IF function, particularly if you want to exercise while doing it.

Have a look at what the experts had to suggest on how to exercise when fasting comfortably and efficiently.

11.1 Getting in a good gym session while fasting

If you choose to try intermittent fasting while continuing to exercise, there are a few things you can really do to make your exercise more successful.

1. Make a schedule

When it comes to getting the workout more successful when fasting, registered dietician Christopher Shuff stated that there are three things to consider: whether you can exercise before, during, or even after the fueling window.

The 16:8 protocol is a common IF form. The idea entails eating everything during an 8-hour fueling timeframe before fasting for 16 hours.

"Working out before the window is best for someone who does well during exercise on an empty stomach, and working out during the window is great for someone who doesn't want to exercise on an empty stomach but needs to take advantage of post-workout nutrition," he says. During is the safest choice for success and regeneration, according to Shuff.

He continues, "After the window is for those who want to work out after fueling but don't have time to do so during the feeding window."

2. Based on the macros, determine the kind of exercise you can do

Lynda Lippin, a certified personal trainer & master pilates instructor, says it's essential to give attention to the macronutrients you consume the day before and after your workout.

Strength workouts, for example, necessitate further carbs on the day of the exercise, while cardio/high-intensity interval training (HIIT) may be performed on a lower carb day, she describes.

3. To develop or sustain strength, eat the right foods during the exercise

According to Dr. Niket Sonpal, the easiest way to combine IF and fitness is to schedule your exercises during your eating cycles so that your nutrition levels are at their highest.

"It's also essential for your body to have protein after a heavy lifting exercise to help in regeneration," he continues.

Following some strength exercise, Amengual recommends eating carbs and around 20 grams of protein within 30 minutes of the workout.

11.2 How do you exercise comfortably while fasting?

Any weight reduction or fitness program's effectiveness is determined by how safe it is to maintain over time. Keep in the safe zone if your ultimate target is to lose body fat and preserve your health level when doing IF. Here are few professional suggestions to assist you in doing so.

1. Closely follow the mild- to high-intensity exercise with a meal

This is when the importance of meal planning falls into action. It's crucial, according to Khorana, to eat prior to a low- or high-intensity exercise. As a result, the body may have some glycogen reserves to draw from to power your exercise.

2. Keep yourself hydrated

It's important to note that fasting does not imply dehydration, according to Sonpal. In reality, he advises drinking more water when fasting.

3. Maintain a healthy electrolyte balance

Coconut water, according to Sonpal, is a healthy, low-calorie hydration source. He claims that it replenishes electrolytes, low in calories, and tastes nice. Stop consuming too much Gatorade or athletic beverages since they are rich in sugar.

4. Maintain a low level of intensity and duration

Take a rest if you feel dizzy or light-headed after pushing yourself so hard. It's important to pay attention to the body.

Think of the kind of quick you'll be doing.

If you are doing a 24-h intermittent fast, Lippin recommends doing low-intensity exercises like:

- Jogging/Walking

- Yoga for relaxation

- Pilates is a gentle workout.

However, since most of the 16-hour fasting window is spent in the evening, sleeping, and early in the morning if you're doing the 16:8 fast, keeping to a certain form of workout isn't as essential.

11.3 Pay attention to the body's signals.

When exercising during IF, the most important thing to remember is to listen to your body. "If you begin to feel tired or dizzy, it's likely that you have low blood sugar or are dehydrated," Amengual says. If that's the case, she recommends starting with a carbohydrate-electrolyte drink and then eating a well-balanced lunch.

Although exercising & intermittent fasting can be beneficial to certain individuals, others may be uncomfortable exercising at all while fasting.

Before beginning any diet or exercise routine, consult the doctor or healthcare professional.

Chapter: 12 Intermittent Fasting and Weight Loss

12.1 Is IF Helpful for Weight Loss?

Have you ever asked if intermittent fasting would help weight loss? The response isn't that cut-and-dry. Fasting is when you don't eat for a long period of time. Intermittent fasting is a straightforward eating practice that utilizes the body's natural fat-burning mechanisms. Intermittent fasting has been shown in studies to help people maintain healthy body weight.

There are many ways to weight reduction, so we're here to discuss weight control, which entails making dietary changes to maintain a healthy weight. Consider intermittent fasting as another weapon in the fitness collection. Continue reading to learn more about the research behind intermittent fasting & weight loss, as well as how to make the most of your quick.

12.2 How does IF affects Weight Management?

Intermittent fasting entails eating all of the food the body requires in a shorter amount of time. There are many approaches, but the most popular is to feed for six to eight hours and then fast for the remaining 14 - 16 hours. It's not nearly as terrible as it looks, particularly if you fuel up with Bulletproof Coffee beforehand to hold hunger at bay.

Intermittent fasting has been shown in several trials to help people lose weight. In a 2015 study of 40 trials, participants lost an average of 10 pounds during a 10-week cycle. Another smaller research found that 16 obese adults who followed an "alternate day" intermittent fasting schedule (consuming 25% of their regular calories on one day and eating normally the next) lost up to 13 pounds in 8 weeks.

Intermittent fasting often causes a confluence of metabolic changes that help with weight loss and management. Here's how it will assist you with maintaining a healthier weight:

1. Calorie Intake is reduced

Whether you snack or consume on the go, you could be consuming more calories than your body requires—and an unhealthy caloric consumption may eventually show up on the scale. When you minimize the period of time you have to consume during the day, you prefer to eat fewer calories.

2. Kickstarts the Ketosis Process

Intermittent fasting is a way to get through ketosis, a fat-burning condition. During a fast, the body uses up its glucose stores (also known as carbohydrates) for energy. You finally start burning dietary and body fat for food if you stay fasted long enough. Eat a ketogenic diet in between fasting cycles to remain in ketosis.

3. Insulin Levels are reduced

Insulin is affected in two forms by intermittent fasting. First, the body becomes more insulin-sensitive, which will help you avoid weight gain and lower the diabetes risk. Second, fasting lowers insulin levels, signalling the body to begin burning accumulated fat rather than glucose.

4. Improves Metabolism

Intermittent fasting reconfigured metabolic processes in rodents, allowing them to get more energy from food.

Fasting has also been found to raise adrenaline and noradrenaline levels. During a short, these hormones assist the body in using stored energy (body fat). Increasing your appetite allows you to burn more calories during the day, including while you are sleeping.

5. Visceral Fat is Target

Intermittent fasting also fails when all other weight-loss programs fall short: it targets and reduces visceral fat. Internal fat wrapped deep around the stomach organs is known as visceral fat. Intermittent fasting diet participants shed 4-7 % of their visceral fat over the course of six months.

6. Inflammation is Reduced

Intermittent fasting reduces oxidative stress and inflammation in general, as well as inflammatory markers like leptin, adiponectin, and (BDNF) brain-derived neurotrophic factor.

Reduced inflammation could be the secret to keeping a safe body weight, increasing longevity, and reducing the likelihood of serious illnesses, according to the initial report (read: rat trials and limited human sample sizes).

12.3 Guidelines for IF Weight Management

You should expect to go through an adjustment period regardless of the intermittent fasting schedule you use— especially if you're used to long meal times that require several meals and snacks. Here are few guidelines to help you control your cravings and stay on track through your fast. During your meal times, enjoy a nutritious diet and start monitoring your food consumption to ensure you're meeting your calorie and macronutrient goals.

1. Get the Right Fats in your diet

Bulletproof Brain Octane, MCT Oil will help you get more energy in your body before you launch your quick. MCTs are converted by your body into ketones, which boost fat burning, reduce cravings, and provide more energy to your brain for improved mental function.

Don't know where to start with MCT oil? It's delicious in Bulletproof Coffee, but it's also delicious in smoothies, salad dressings, and dips like this guacamole. Who doesn't like the healthier fats of avocados in a decent guacamole recipe?

2. Carbs can be reduced

Reduce your carb intake (whole grains, starches, and sugars) during your feeding window to maximize the advantages of intermittent fasting. Reduce your appetite (bye-bye, energy crashes) and making things easier for your body, move into fat-burning ketosis by eating more high-quality fats and limiting carbohydrates.

If you are not able to go all-in on keto, consider low carb diet instead they are not the same.

3. Meals can be planned ahead of time

When it's time to feed, some sweets & snacks seem really tempting. Prepare nutritious meals ahead of time with the correct fats, high-quality meats, and lots of salads to prevent bingeing on carbs or junk food. You'll be able to keep on board with these keto meal planning recipes.

12.4 Weight Lose Faster by Exercising on an Empty Stomach

Have you ever been advised to exercise with an empty stomach? Fasted cardio, or cardio performed before or after eating, is a common subject in the health and diet world.

There are supporters and detractors, as with many wellness phenomena. Some people swear it's a quick and easy way to lose weight, while others think it's a waste of time and effort.

Fasted cardio doesn't often imply that you're doing an intermittent fasting plan. It could be as easy as going for a morning run and then enjoying breakfast.

12.5 Fitness & Nutrition Experts Suggestion

The benefits and drawbacks of fasted cardio were discussed with three health and diet experts. This is what they have to suggest about it.

1. Do it; Fasted cardio will help you lose more calories and fat

In weight loss and exercise circles, going for a workout session on the upright cycle or treadmill before eating is popular. The prospect of burning more fat is often the primary motivator. So how does it work in practice?

Emmie Satrazemis, CSSD, RD, a board-certified sports nutritionist & nutrition director at Trifecta, says, "Not getting extra calories or food on hand from a latest meal or before the snack forces the body to focus on retained fuel, which occurs to be glycogen and stored fat."

She mentions a few small studies that claim that working out in the morning after a fast of 8 to 12 hours when sleeping will help you burn up to 20% more fat. However, several reports have shown that it has little impact on total fat loss.

2. Skip it; If you want to gain muscle mass, you must eat before a cardio workout

However, there is a distinction to be made between gaining muscle mass and maintaining muscle mass.

"As long as you consume enough protein and use your muscles, research shows that muscle mass is very well protected and in a calorie deficit," Satrazemis explains.

That's because amino acids are not as attractive as stored carbohydrates and fat while your body is searching for food. Satrazemis, on the other hand, claims that the supply of instant energy is limited and that exercising too hard for too long when fasting can cause you to run out of gas or begin to break down more muscle.

She also claims that eating after a workout helps you to replenish these stores as well as restore the muscle damage that happened during your workout.

3. Do it; You like the way fasted cardio makes your body feel

This explanation can seem self-evident, but it is not unusual to wonder why we do things, even though they make us happy. As a result, Satrazemis believes that the choice to pursue fasted cardio is a personal one. "Some people like to exercise on an empty stomach, while others do best while they eat," she explains.

4. Skip it; Activities that necessitate a lot of strength and pace can be done with food in the stomach

According to David Chesworth (ACSM-certified personal trainer), if you intend on doing an exercise that requires high levels of strength or speed, you can eat before doing certain exercises.

He explains why glucose is the best fuel for strength and speed operations since it is the fastest type of energy. "The physiology does not usually provide the optimal tools for this form of exercise in a fasted state," Chesworth notes. As a result, if you want to get quick and strong, he recommends training after eating.

5. Do it; If you have GI stress, Fasted cardio can be beneficial

If you eat a meal or even a snack before performing the exercise, you can feel sick throughout your workout. "This is particularly true in the morning, as well as with high fat and high fiber foods," Satrazemis says.

If you can't afford a bigger meal or don't have at least 2 days to process it, you could be best served eating anything with a simple energy supply — or doing exercise when fasted.

6. Skip it; You have several health issues

You must be in outstanding shape to do cardio in a fasted condition. You can also remember health issues like low blood sugar or low blood pressure, which may induce dizziness and place you at risk for injuries, according to Satrazemis.

12.6 Tips for Performing Fasted Cardio

If you wish to attempt fasted cardio, keep the following guidelines in mind to ensure your safety:

- If you don't eat, don't do more than 60 minutes of cardio.

- Choose exercises that are mild to low-intensity.

- Drinking water is a part of fasted cardio, so remain hydrated.

- Keep in mind that your overall lifestyle, especially your diet, has a greater impact on your weight gain or loss than the frequency of your workouts.

Pay attention to health and do what feels right. If you're unsure whether or not you can perform fasted cardio, seek advice from a registered nutritionist, personal trainer, or doctor.

Chapter: 13 Intermittent Fasting and Supplements

Intermittent fasting increases concentration, burns body fat, and puts the aging process on the back burner. Fasting includes going without calories for a period of time, so what about supplements? Fasting supplements will also help the body burn fat for food, which might sound counterintuitive.

So, if you're fasting, will you take supplements? It is based on the situation. Here are the details on which nutritional supplements to take and which to not, as well as the science behind how it all operates.

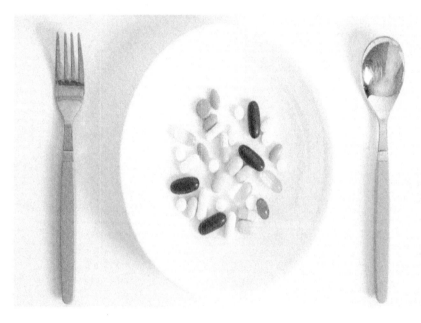

13.1 Supplements to take during a Fast

All intermittent fasting supplements can be used on an empty stomach to avoid breaking a fast. Pay attention to the emotions. Some people are unable to take vitamins without consuming food. If that's the case, consider taking them 20 to 30 minutes before your dinner.

1. Creatine

If you take it before or during a workout, creatine provides no calories and has no effect on insulin levels, so it won't break the fast.

2. Electrolytes

Potassium, sodium, and calcium are examples of electrolytes. It is good to take an electrolyte substitute after a quick as long as it doesn't have any calories or sweeteners, and it may also help you handle the side effects of converting to ketosis.

3. L-tyrosine

Don't worry—safe it's to take this on an empty stomach. L-tyrosine may help in tension control and mood support. While it is an amino acid, it is unlikely to crack quickly when consumed in small quantities.

4. Probiotics

Probiotics are helpful microbes that live in your stomach, and having a healthy gut protects your whole body. When stomach acid levels are down, certain probiotic supplements may be taken without eating. The manufacturer's instructions can be found on the packaging of your probiotic replacement.

5. Prebiotics

Probiotics need food, and Prebiotics provide food for the good gut bacteria, which helps to maintain a stable gut microbiome. Bulletproof Inner Fuel Prebiotic has no sugar and no net carbs, and it dissolves quickly in hot or cold liquids. In the morning, try it with a cup of black coffee.

6. Water-soluble Vitamins

During a fasting time, you should take vitamins B & C with water. On an empty stomach, vitamin C is normally simple to take, but B-complex vitamins can cause people to feel nauseous if taken without food. If this happens to you, simply break your fast and take these vitamins.

13.2 Supplements to take with food

A few of these supplements are better consumed when taken with food. Others can break your fast, but save them until when you can feed.

1. Amino Acid

Branched-chain amino acids (BCAAs) and L-glutamine are typically avoided during fasting because they will trigger insulin levels to rise, causing you to exit ketosis.

2. Curcumin & Omega-3 fatty acids

When consumed with fruit, supplements including Bulletproof Omega Krill Complex and Bulletproof Curcumin Max are better to consume. As a result, consume them across the eating window.

3. Vanadium & Chromium

When fasting, these minerals will cause the blood sugar levels to drop too much. Hypoglycemia, with low blood sugar and low energy levels, will occur if the insulin levels drop. However, a minor case of hypoglycemia will make it difficult to change and manage your moods. When you're ready to break your high, take these supplements.

4. Fat-Soluble Vitamins

Vitamin E, vitamin D, and multivitamins with fat-soluble components also fall under this group. Since these vitamins do not dissolve in water, they must be taken with food. Check the label for instructions if you're not sure. Take one soft gel every day with food, according to Bulletproof Vitamins A-D-K.

5. Gummy Vitamins

Gummy vitamins are sweetened and filled with gelatin, which includes protein, so they'll most certainly break a fast.

6. Iodine

Take the potassium iodide tablets or kelp powder with food for optimum absorption.

7. Magnesium

After taking a magnesium supplement on empty stomach, certain people can feel stomach discomfort.

8. Protein Powder

If it's whey or collagen protein, either protein powder includes calories and activates an insulin reaction, so it breaks quickly. So, reserve the protein powder while you're feeding.

9. Zins & Copper

Zinc and copper are two minerals that fit well together, but you will also find them in pill shape together. With food, take Bulletproof Zinc with Copper.

13.3 Science behind Fasting Supplements

You can stop eating something that violates your fast if you want to gain the most health benefits from intermittent fasting. Any calorie-dense foods or liquids, as well as supplements that stimulate digestion or raise insulin levels, fall under this category.

This is why:

- Autophagy, the mechanism by which the cells get rid of built-up garbage, is triggered when you go without food for long periods of time.

- Fasting encourages the body to undergo ketosis, a physiological condition in which fat is burned for fuel. To work, the body requires energy. When you miss meals, the body uses up the accumulated glucose (from carbohydrates) before turning to fat for nutrition.

- Fasting will also allow your body to produce a protein known as (FIAF) stands for fasting-induced adipose factor, that tells your body that it's time to start burning fat.

To summarise, you can use caution while supplementing since some of them can split your fast and allow you to exit ketosis. Others won't break your soon, but they shouldn't be consumed on an empty stomach.

What's the big deal with that? If you take a vitamin without eating, it can move through the body without being fully consumed. Others can make you feel sick if you take them with an empty stomach. Thank you, just no.

Warning: If you take prescribed drugs, consult a doctor before changing your supplementation plan. Any prescriptions may be administered within a certain amount of time. Others can experience side effects if they are taken on an empty stomach.

13.4 What about drinks as Tea, Coffee & Bone Broth?

While both unsweetened tea and black coffee have calories, the number is small (less than 5 calories) and unlikely to ruin your quick. Stick to water if you're a fasting purist. Tea and coffee are also acceptable sources of caffeine.

Since it's a relaxing way to replenish minerals and nutrients during a fast, bone broth is a common keto fasting supplement. It contains very little calories, protein, and carbohydrates, but even a tiny quantity won't significantly alter the ketogenic or fat-burning advantages of fasting. Save all the bone broth for your feeding window if you choose to optimize autophagy.

Bottom Line

The bottom line is that you should take vitamins while fasting. Taking the supplements and medications through your feeding window, whether they disturb your stomach and need to be taken with meals. Experiment to see what is well for you and what makes you happy.

Chapter: 14 Top 5 Supplements for Intermittent Fasting

It may be difficult to maintain a healthy diet that provides all of the essential nutrients. Nutritionists and Dietitians, after all, spend years on how to navigate our nutrition and diets.

Intermittent fasting adds another layer of difficulty to the equation. You are going to miss any vital nutrients and minerals if you have limited eating time.

Intermittent fasting supplements can be useful in this situation. Some vitamins can help you avoid nutritional shortages, and others can help you move your intermittent fasting to the next stage.

Here are five intermittent fasting supplements to think about if you are fasting:

1. Multivitamin
2. Probiotics
3. Electrolytes
4. BCAA
5. MCT oil

Let's have a deeper look at why these nutrients are so essential and how to integrate them into your fasting routine.

14.1 Multivitamin

1. What Do Multivitamins Do?

Multivitamin supplements are composed of many different minerals and vitamins, as well as other components. This supplement is used to boost vitamins that you don't get from your food.

According to a new nationwide study in the United States, 94 percent of the population were deficient in vitamin D, 88 percent in vitamin E, and 43 percent in vitamin A. Unless you eat a well-balanced intermittent fasting diet, it's obvious that you're not getting enough antioxidants from food alone.

If you are doing a fasting routine that allows you to fast for the whole day, such as OMAD fasting or prolonged & extended fasting with fasts longer than 24 hours, multivitamin supplements are strongly suggested.

2. How to Take Multivitamins?

Multivitamin supplements are usually taken during the eating window. Multivitamins contain fat-soluble vitamins including A, D, E and K, which can be taken with food.

It does not matter whether it is dinner, lunch or breakfast; the diet can have some good fat because it helps the body's absorption of fat-soluble vitamins. Another advantage is that drinking a multivitamin after a meal reduces the possibility of stomach problems or nausea from these nutrients.

3. Which Multivitamin Is Best for Fasting?

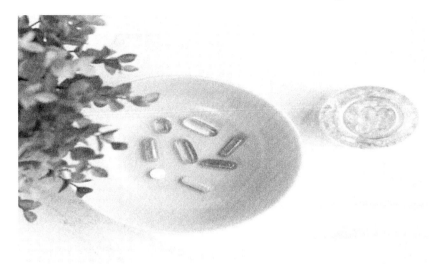

For intermittent fasting, any high-quality multivitamin would suffice. Artificial colors, titanium dioxide, and carrageenan can also be avoided. Check to see whether the Multivitamin has any of the most often lacking vitamins and minerals, such as magnesium, vitamin D, zinc, calcium and iron for women.

You should also search for multivitamins that are formulated for the specific demographic, such as multivitamins for men over 50 or multivitamins for women.

14.2 Probiotics

1. What Do Probiotics Do?

Bacteria aren't always made equal. There are trillions of microbes on or in humans, with our gut accounted for more than 80% of them. Probiotics are live bacteria that help us synthesize vitamins and digest fiber. According to recent research, bacterial imbalances in the intestine may have a negative effect on our mental health.

Probiotics are live bacteria that can be contained in fermented foods like yogurt, sauerkraut, kimchi, miso & kefir. They're called "healthy" bacteria because they help with digestion and inflammation.

If you don't have foods high in probiotics in your intermittent fasting diet, you may be having intestinal problems like constipation, diarrhea, or bloating. Since not everybody loves probiotic-rich diets, probiotic extracts may be used as an alternative.

2. How to Take Probiotics?

Many probiotic supplement manufacturers advocate having it on an empty stomach, although others recommend taking it with food. As a result, it is dependent on the specific probiotic supplement.

You should eat it during the quick if it's recommended to have it on an empty stomach. Otherwise, you should take your probiotic supplements for every meal.

3. Which Probiotics Is Best for Fasting?

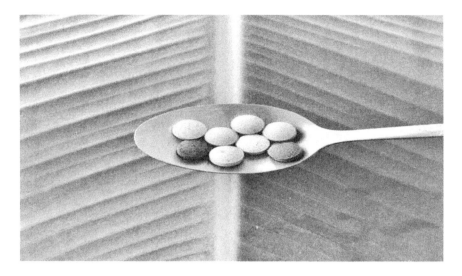

Your probiotic can be as complex as your stomach. One probiotic strain can be used in the cheapest probiotics. Look for a supplement that includes several probiotic strains to get the most benefits.

14.3 Electrolytes

1. What Do Electrolytes Do?

Electrolytes are minerals that are essential for life, such as calcium, magnesium, sodium and potassium. They are important in assisting the body in a variety of tasks, including energy production, water regulation, muscle control, and metabolism.

Many of the essential electrolytes can be obtained from a well-balanced diet. You could be at risk of electrolyte shortage if you restrict your food or feeding hours. Fatigue, headaches, nausea, and muscle cramps are also possible side effects. Another incentive to review your intermittent fasting plan or go for a carefully designed intermittent fasting meal schedule to guarantee you receive enough of the nutrients you need.

Electrolytes are often discussed in relation to dehydration and are listed in advertisements for sports drinks since they are primarily lost by sweat and urine. If you exercise daily and limit your food consumption with extended fasting, electrolyte supplements can be beneficial. You will maintain a healthy electrolyte balance in the body this way.

2. How to Take Electrolytes?

Electrolytes can be consumed on empty stomach and are calorie-free. As a result, you will consume electrolytes during the fasting period. This supplement will not cause you to break your early.

This is true with electrolyte tablets, which we use if you're searching for a supplement to replenish the electrolytes. Though sports drinks are popular for supplying electrolytes, they also involve a high level of sugar & food coloring. Sports drinks are not the healthiest choice, and they will undoubtedly break yours soon.

3. Which Electrolytes are Best for Fasting?

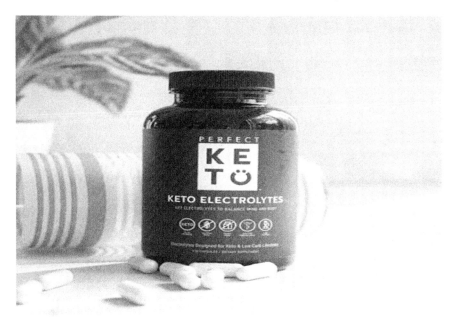

Above ideal, Keto Electrolyte capsules are my top pick. These include magnesium, calcium, sodium, and potassium, which are four of the most important electrolytes lost during intermittent fasting and exercise.

Perfect Keto has a variety of intermittent fasting-friendly options and always mentions whether or not you should use the food without stopping your fast. For example, they've ensured that these Electrolyte capsules can be comfortably consumed on an empty stomach and during the fasting window.

14.4 BCAA

1. What Do BCCA Do?

BCaas stands for (Branched-Chain Amino Acids) are a group of three basic amino acids that are particularly beneficial to our muscles. Such amino acids are needed for your body to regenerate and develop new muscle.

Since the body cannot produce BCAAs, we must obtain them from our diet. Meat, dairy, egg, poultry, and fish are all good sources of BCAAs. In most cases, a well-balanced diet would include all of the necessary amino acids needed for muscle growth.

However, since keeping to a short eating window makes it difficult to ingest the same volume of food, you will not be able to recharge BCAAs as easily. It's especially necessary when intermittent fasting & exercise are combined. BCAA supplementation may help muscle development, minimize exercise exhaustion, and reduce post-workout soreness.

2. How to Take BCCA?

BCAAs provide both protein and calories, so eating them during the fasting window can result in a break in the fast. It's better to get your BCAAs within the eating time if you're on a strict fast.

If you're doing a lot of exercises, want to build muscle, or are continually tired during workouts, you may want to try taking BCAA supplements during fasting. After all, it's crucial to pay attention to your health, so if a BCAA shake helping you get through your exercises and achieve your goals, go for it. The advantages of BCAAs for your exercise can outweigh the risks of technically breaking the hard.

3.   Which BCCA is Best for Fasting?

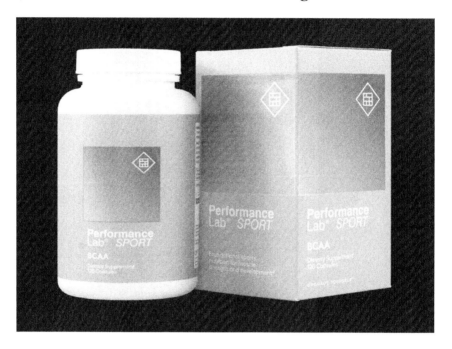

Seek BCAA supplements that are free of colorants, preservatives, and other ingredients. Performance Lab BCAA capsules are my preferred BCAA for intermittent fasting since they are the easiest. To block the taste of BCAAs, most BCAA powders produce artificial flavors and sweeteners. Capsules, on the other side, are tasteless and odorless.

14.5 MCT Oil

1. What Does it Do?

MCT stands for (medium-chain triglycerides) oil is made from a form of fat present in dairy products as well as oils such as coconut and palm oil. It's a well-known weight-loss and energy-boosting supplement.

"How does oil benefit with fat loss?" you may wonder. Ketosis is the solution. Your body will enter a state known as ketosis with the support of intermittent fasting or the keto diet. That's where the body switches from using glucose from carbohydrates to using ketones, which are produced from fat. As a result, once you've reached the fat-burning stage of ketosis, MCT oil can just provide more fuel to your bloodstream, not kick you out.

MCT oil has been seen in studies to fill people up quicker, resulting in them consuming fewer overall. You will hold the body in ketosis and begin to burn fat, thus curbing your appetite.

2. How to Use MCT Oil?

MCT oil is made up entirely of fat, which ensures it is high in calories. Using MCT oil during the fasting window would then cause the fast to be broken.

Breaking your quick with bulletproof coffee is the most effective way to use MCT oil:

1 cup coffee, 1 to 2 tablespoons MCT oil, & 1 to 2 tablespoons unsalted grass-fed butter or ghee. Blend the products for 30 seconds or before they resemble a smooth latte. Enjoy your MCT oil coffee, which is both filling and energizing. This coffee will hold you in ketosis for a couple more hours, allowing you to continue burning fat.

Another choice is to incorporate MCT oil into your meals at mealtime. MCT oil shakes & smoothies are another excellent way to incorporate them into the diet. Just keep in mind that it's a high-calorie snack; even if you're not on a keto diet, these all calories might not contribute to weight loss.

3. Which is the Best MCT Oil for Fasting?

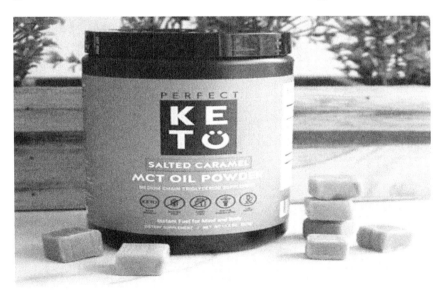

When it comes to intermittent fasting or Keto, its needed to bring attention to the best MCT oils. MCT oil in powder shape was my preference. It produces the creamiest bulletproof coffee & doesn't trigger stomach upset, which is a typical side effect of MCT oil.

The favorite is Perfect Keto MCT powder, which comes in five flavors: vanilla, chocolate, matcha latte, salted caramel and unflavoured. Almond milk can be transformed into fluffy chocolate milk with the addition of the chocolate one. This MCT oil is also one of the purest I've seen, with no added sweeteners or potentially dangerous additives.

Which Supplement Can You Use for Intermittent Fasting?

Intermittent fasting may take several forms, varying from the less restrictive 18/6 to extended fasting or even dry fasting. Multiple types of intermittent fasting will necessitate various supplements:

- When doing extended fasting or having dietary requirements that exclude some food groups, multivitamins, electrolytes, and probiotics are particularly recommended.

- If you frequently exercise when fasting intermittently, you should recommend taking a BCAA, electrolyte, and MCT oil supplement. These intermittent fasting supplements can help you stay energized for your workouts while still allowing you to heal quickly.

- If you are a fan of Keto or intermittent fasting, MCT oil will help you get more fat and electrolytes while avoiding the keto flu.

The path to your ideal body weight would be much easier if you have the correct intermittent fasting vitamins on hand. Check out the 21 Days of Intermittent Fasting Challenge if you haven't tried intermittent fasting yet or aren't sure where to go. It also provides a nutritious meal schedule to ensure that the body has all of the required macro and micronutrients.

Chapter: 15 Pros and Cons of Intermittent Fasting

Although promising research on the potential effects of intermittent fasting exists, much of the health claims are focused on animal experiments. Although there are a few human experiments on intermittent fasting, the findings are sometimes contradictory. In order to get a better understanding of the possible health benefits of intermittent fasting, more comprehensive human testing is needed.

But, what would the research mean about intermittent fasting & its health effects? Let's dig at the benefits and drawbacks of intermittent fasting.

15.1 Pros of Intermittent Fasting

1. Weight Loss

Fasting has been attributed to a substantial decrease in body fat, body weight and waist circumference in many human studies. Similarly, a report published in 2020 showed that using intermittent fasting to manage obesity was extremely successful, with participants losing 8-13 percent of their body weight.

In addition, a systematic study and meta-analysis published in 2019 showed that intermittent fasting was only as efficient for weight loss as (CER) Continuous Energy Restriction. As a result, a more relaxed lifestyle, such as extended fasting, will achieve similar weight loss outcomes as a restrictive diet.

2. Fat Loss

In comparison to regular calorie restriction-type diets, studies have shown that intermittent fasting can help boost fat loss while maintaining fat-free mass (aka muscle mass) when combined with adequate protein intake and resistance training.

3. Blood Sugar

Intermittent fasting has been shown in animal research to increase glucose homeostasis and insulin sensitivity. When opposed to a continuous energy restriction diet, intermittent fasting resulted in a lower HbA1C (long-term blood sugar levels), according to a 2017 systematic review.

4. Blood Pressure & Cholesterol

Fasting for short periods of time can help lower LDL and overall cholesterol levels. It has also been found in several studies to lower blood pressure & triglyceride levels. Both of these steps are vital for reducing and preventing the risk of a variety of diseases, including cardiovascular disease.

5. Inflammation

Intermittent fasting has also been attributed to a decrease in inflammation in the body. Intermittent fasting has been shown to improve adiponectin levels and may help to reduce inflammation by inhibiting inflammation-causing monocytes.

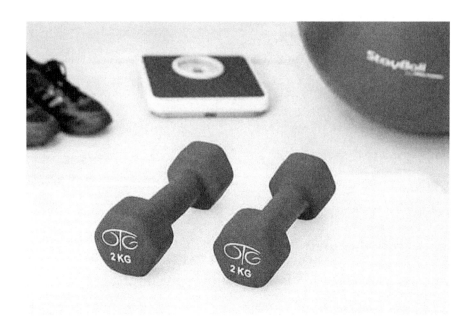

6. Brain Functioning

In a 2018 study, intermittent fasting was linked to lower oxidative stress and improved memory. It was also found that prolonged fasting was linked to a longer lifespan and a lower risk of age-related diseases. Almost all of the research in the study, though, was done on animals.

7. No Calorie Limits

Yes, that is right! You don't have to reduce your regular calorie intake or adjust the types of foods you consume. In terms of short-term weight reduction, studies have shown no significant gap between continuous calorie restriction and fasting.

8. Larger Servings in a Shorter Timeframe

Since eating greater portions of food in one sitting help fit with your normal appetite and fullness signals, some people may choose the shorter eating window during intermittent fasting. Intermittent fasting, on the other hand, can be more difficult to stick to for those who enjoy smaller, more regular meals during the day.

15.2 Cons of Intermittent Fasting

1. Interferes with Eating Social Aspects

Eating is a social activity to a certain extent. All of our gatherings, milestones, and special events revolve around food if you think about it. Intermittent fasting, on the other hand, can make social gatherings around food difficult due to the shortened eating window.

Not to mention the late-night romantic meals, home-cooked family suppers, wedding dinners, lunch sessions with your employer and co-workers, and maybe even share a meal with your wife and kids. Not a lot of entertainment.

2. Low Energy Levels

According to a systematic review published in 2016, certain intermittent fasting users reported mild physical side effects such as coldness, constipation, headaches, exhaustion, bad temper, and lack of concentration. It will be challenging to find the desire or inspiration to be involved and go through your everyday life under these circumstances.

It's important to have enough fuel during the day to keep our energy levels up. With that in mind, certain people can find intermittent fasting difficult if adhering to a time-restricted eating plan interferes with their everyday activities & hunger levels. This leads us to our next step...

3. Increase in Human Hunger

If intermittent fasting causes an uncomfortable level of hunger, it's possible that certain people would eat more than they usually will when their eating window actually opens up. Although intermittent fasting may work for some people without increasing hunger, it all comes down to your personal hunger & fullness cues.

If you get hungry later in the day and are more comfortable with three larger meals, intermittent fasting might be a better fit for you. However, if you want to eat smaller, more regular meals during the day and are hungry throughout the morning and at night, intermittent fasting can make you feel even more hungry throughout the fasting windows.

4. Digestive Problems

After eating a significant quantity of food in one sitting within their eating windows, certain people can feel digestive pain. Gas, cramping, stomach discomfort, indigestion, and bloating are examples of digestive symptoms. However, since each person's body is different, whether or not you develop digestive problems as a result of intermittent fasting is extremely individualized. This is something to consider if intermittent fasting significantly changes the eating habits or the volume of food you consume in one sitting.

Individuals with IBS, on the other hand, might not be a suitable match for intermittent fasting since their guts are more sensitive and resistant to inflammation. As a result, these people are more prone to cramping, stomach pain, and bloating.

5. Effect on Heart Health is Uncertain

Intermittent fasting on alternating days provided mixed results for cardiovascular indicators like total cholesterol. Both LDL & HDL (BAD cholesterol & GOOD cholesterol) rates had increased in this research, while triglyceride levels decreased. Other tests, on the other hand, indicate that overall cholesterol and LDL levels decreased while HDL levels remained unchanged. Given the mixed results, further human trials on intermittent fasting are obviously needed to get a better understanding of its effect on heart health.

6. Disordered eating may trigger

Intermittent fasting could be triggering if you have a background of disordered eating or an eating disorder, and it is not advisable for you. Following a collection of "laws" during intermittent fasting (when it's appropriate to eat and when it's not) may interfere with your relationship with food rather than listening to your internal hunger cues.

As previously mentioned, it could trigger increased hunger, which may contribute to a binge, exacerbating chronic eating disorder symptoms or reinforcing the "binge-restrict" mentality. In addition, a 2016 study discovered that certain intermittent fasting users have a diet addiction.

7. Long Term Health Consequences for Women

About the fact that intermittent fasting does not explicitly require food restriction (because there is no caloric restriction during eating windows), it can lead to calorie reduction.

With this in mind, limiting energy and protein too much may contribute to nutritional deficiencies, which can lead to problems with fertility and reproduction in women.

Fasting decreased blood glucose levels, body weight and, most surprisingly, ovary size, both of which had a major effect on fertility in rats, according to several animal research. The luteinizing hormone, which regulates ovulation, was shown to be impaired by three consecutive days of complete fasting during the mid-follicular stages, according to a 2017 study on women. It has little impact on follicle growth or the duration of the menstrual cycle.

While there are little human researches on the effects of intermittent fasting on fertility, these important findings indicate that human females may experience similar effects.

8. Weight Gain Potential

If you reduce your energy consumption too dramatically, your body can react with physiological adaptations. And the fact that intermittent fasting would not limit daily calories, the time-restricted eating windows often contribute to weight gain.

That said, any dramatic weight loss (whether from intermittent fasting or another restrictive diet) will lead to weight gain – a condition known as weight cycling.

In any event, it's impossible to say if intermittent fasting, in particular, causes weight gain, and there haven't been any long-term trials to see whether the diet is effective.

9. Metabolism is Slower

When you fast for long stretches of time without eating enough calories, your body goes into starvation mode. When you're hungry, your metabolism slows down to save resources, and your body starts using muscle protein as a source of food. Even a 24-hour quick will reduce the BMR (Basal Metabolic Rate).

Chapter 16: 7-Day Intermittent Fasting Meal Plan

We designed a 7-Day Intermittent Fasting Plan to help you get started on your Intermittent Fasting journey in a simple, enjoyable, and sustainable manner. It includes an activity for each day, as well as concise overview & additional learnings.

Scroll down to have a brief look at the seven days of Intermittent Fasting. If you believe it's time to regain control of your health and make Intermittent Fasting a way of life, let's go.

FIRST WEEK DAILY PLAN

Day 1	Day 2	Day 3	Day 4	Day 5	Day 6	Day 7
12H FAST 12H EAT	13H FAST 11H EAT	14H FAST 10H EAT	15H FAST 9H EAT	16H FAST 8H EAT	16H FAST 8H EAT	16H FAST 8H EAT
START & pick your Intermittent Fasting schedule	Learn the basics of Intermittent Fasting	Define your rewards	Prepare a high protein lunch	Drink black coffee when hungry	Go for a walk	Reflect on your progress

1. DAY First

* **Task:** 12 hour Fast & 12 hour Eat

* **Mission:** Select your IF Schedule

You can gradually ease into intermittent fasting over the first week. This is why we recommend beginning with 12 hours of fasting on the first day and gradually growing to 16 hours on Day 5 by adding 1 hour per day. It would be better for the body and brain to adjust to the new eating pattern this way, and you will have more flexibility to get adjusted to Intermittent Fasting.

We will want you to pick the Intermittent Fasting schedule that better fit your personality. Consistency has been shown to be one of the most important aspects in achieving success.

2. DAY Second

- **Task:** 13 hour Fast & 11 hour Eat
- **Mission:** Learn about the fundamentals of intermittent fasting

Your fast will be extended to 13 hours on Day 2. You have one hour more than yesterday – you should do it.

Day 2 is a wonderful day to start learning about healthier eating habits that can help you achieve your Intermittent Fasting targets: just concentrate on eating more whole foods while avoiding the normal suspects, including sugar, unhealthy foods, & empty carbs.

We will give you a list of popular meals and foods that you should consume to improve your Intermittent Fasting outcomes. Consider plain, tasty, and well-balanced home-cooked meals like meatballs with zucchini noodles, poached eggs with spinach, homemade hummus for a snack or feta cheese salad.

3. DAY Third

- **Task:** 14 hour Fast & 10 hour Eat
- **Mission:** Explain the rewards

When it comes to designing a new Intermittent Fasting pattern, rewards are important. As a result, on Day 3, we want you to determine your own incentives for each day you quickly successfully.

Why is it so necessary to be rewarded?

A reward sends a signal to the brain that says, "This feels amazing, so let's do more of it!" Something that makes you happy, maybe it.

Intermittent Fasting rewards can ideally be linked to your basic needs for relaxation, socialization, sleep, or play.

Alternatively, the incentive may be a quick (but powerful!) celebratory gesture such as cheering yourself up & saying "Good work" or crossing another day off of the daily success monitoring sheet you received when you joined the task.

If the incentive is more significant, such as a meal at an expensive yet delicious restaurant, you may use the token strategy, in which each good day of fasting "gives you" one token. You will treat yourself to a meal at the restaurant until you have received 5 tokens.

4. **DAY Four**

- **Task:** 15 hours Fast & 9 hour Eat

- **Mission:** Make lunch with a lot of protein

You will have also fasted for 15 hours on Day 4 of Intermittent Fasting. We suggest a high-protein lunch to help you split your fast and achieve your weight-loss goals.

You may, for example, make steamed or grilled vegetables with your favorite protein, such as grilled beef, seafood, poultry, tofu, eggs, legumes, beans, nuts, and seeds.

5. DAY Five

- **Task:** 16 hour Fast & 8 hour Eat
- **Mission:** Take black coffee when hungry

You can successfully hit the ultimate 16/8 Intermittent Fasting regimen of fasting for 16 hours and eating during an 8-hour timeframe on Day 5 of the Intermittent Fasting Plan, and that would be relatively simple to do, as we have demonstrated in ourselves and in the hundreds of individuals that have already completed the Intermittent Fasting Task.

We suggest consuming black coffee to help you get through the 16 hours of fasting and to satisfy some hunger you might have. It's high in antioxidants which will help you lose weight (but don't overdo it!).

Keep in mind the coffee for Intermittent Fasting is dark. That is, no sugar, syrup, or creamers can be added to it – no cappuccino, latte, or flat white, just black coffee.

If you must have something delicious, try stevia, a natural sweetener, but be cautious because it can trigger hunger.

Are you a non-coffee drinker? Choose a bottle of water or a cup of black or green tea.

6. DAY Six

- **Task:** 16 hour Fast & 8 hour Eat

- **Mission:** Walk outside

Are you planning to lose weight during fasting? Maintaining a balanced diet is important, and we also suggest doing some exercise in your daily routine.

Well, before you break your fast, go outside for a walk. Even a short 20-minute walk will sufficient.

Walking is an excellent way to increase your physical health, change your outlook, and get some fresh air. Most notably, going on a walk will distract you from your hunger and let the last few hours of fasting fly by faster.

7. DAY Seven

- **Task:** 16 hour Fast & 8 hour Eat

- **Mission:** Go for Walk

Maintain your current 16/8 Intermittent Fasting Schedule today, and focus on your results from the last days.

Taking a full-body snapshot, recording your weight, and comparing them to your starting weight & photo is an important aspect of performance. Your weight and/or outward appearance should start to improve.

In addition, we'd like you to address a few questions about your results, such as how you're doing, whether you've seen any improvements in your energy, attitude, or skin as a result of intermittent fasting, and so on.

Going through such activity will assist you in identifying when and, most specifically, why you might be failing, allowing you to take steps to improve your performance and establish intermittent fasting as a new healthy habit.

Chapter: 17 Salad Recipes

1. Veggie Packed Chicken Cheesy Salad

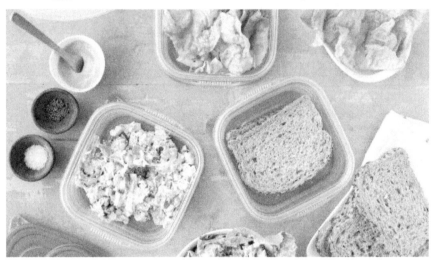

Prep Time	35 mins
Serves	2 persons

NUTRITION INFO

Calories: 364.5	
Calories from Fat 81 g	22 %
Total Fat 9.1 g	13 %
Saturated Fat 3.1 g	15 %
Cholesterol 131.8 mg	43 %
Sodium 767.4 mg	31 %

Total Carbohydrate 15.3 g	5 %
Dietary Fiber 2.8 g	11 %
Sugars 7.3 g	29 %
Protein 53.2 g	106 %

INGREDIENTS

- 1 cup of boneless cooked chicken breast, cubed
- 1⁄2 cup of roughly chopped Baby Spinach
- 1⁄4 cup of chopped celery
- 2 1⁄2 tbsp fat-free mayonnaise
- 1⁄4 cup carrot, crop into ribbons
- 1⁄8 tbsp of dried parsley
- 2 tbsp non-fat sour cream
- 2 teaspoons Dijon mustard
- 1⁄4 cup cheddar cheese, reduced-fat sharp

INSTRUCTIONS

1) In a mixing dish, combine both ingredients and toss well to cover with the mayonnaise mixture.

2) Refrigerate for at least 30 minutes, although it's better if you do it the night before.

2. Sauerkraut Salad

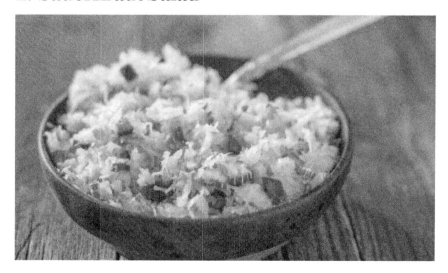

Prep Time	15 mins
Serves	6 persons

NUTRITION INFO

Calories: 224.1	
Calories from Fat 109 g	49 %
Total Fat 12.2 g	18 %
Saturated Fat 1.7 g	8 %
Cholesterol 0 mg	0 %
Sodium 708.5 mg	29 %
Total Carbohydrate 29.7 g	9 %
Dietary Fiber 2.8 g	11 %

Sugars 27.1 g	108 %
Protein 1 g	1 %

INGREDIENTS

- 1 (1 lb) can drained, sauerkraut, but not rinsed
- ½ cup of chopped fine green pepper
- 1 cup of chopped fine celery
- 2 tbsp chopped fine onions
- ½ tbsp salt
- ¾ cup of sugar
- ½ tbsp of pepper
- ⅓ cup salad oil
- ⅓ cup cider, or 1/3 cup vinegar white

INSTRUCTIONS

1) Combine mixed vegetables and sauerkraut in a mixing bowl.

2) Heat the sugar, oil, vinegar, salt, and pepper in a small saucepan over low heat until the sugar has dissolved.

3) Allow to cool before pouring over the vegetables.

4) Allow to chill overnight.

3. Vegetable Roasted Farro Salad

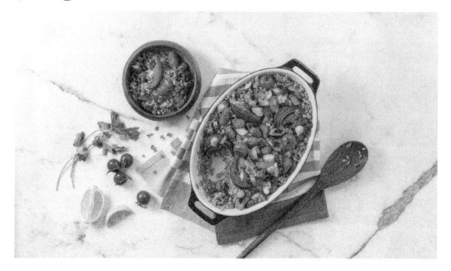

Prep Time	1 hour & 35 mins
Serves	4 persons

NUTRITION INFO

Calories: 123.9	0%
Calories from Fat 75 g	61 %
Total Fat 8.4 g	12 %
Saturated Fat 1.2 g	5 %
Cholesterol 0 mg	0 %
Sodium 2046.5 mg	85 %
Total Carbohydrate 11.5 g	3 %
Dietary Fiber 4 g	15 %

Sugars 5.6 g	22 %
Protein 3 g	5 %

INGREDIENTS

- 1⁄2 medium eggplant, peel on & large diced
- 1 tbsp kosher salt or sea salt
- 1 medium zucchini, peel on & large diced
- 1 cup of washed cherry tomatoes & left whole
- 6 garlic cloves, trimmed peeled and sliced
- 6 white button quartered mushrooms
- 1⁄2 medium onion, peeled & cut into wedges
- 1 tbsp olive oil
- 1 cup of cracked farro
- 2 cups of almond milk
- 1 tbsp of balsamic vinegar
- 1 tbsp of olive oil 15 mL
- 1 tbsp olive oil
- 3 sprigs cilantro
- 1⁄2 tbsp of pepper
- 1⁄2 tbsp salt

INSTRUCTIONS

1) Preheat oven to 425 degrees Fahrenheit (200 degrees Celsius).

2) Salt the eggplant slices thoroughly on both sides in a wide flat pan or baking dish, toss to cover uniformly, and set aside for 30 min to release excess bitterness and moisture.

3) Toss the eggplant into a big mixing bowl after draining and rinsing it. Combine the peppers, zucchini, mushrooms, garlic, and onions in a large mixing bowl. Drizzle olive oil over the vegetables and season with pepper and salt, tossing to coat. Transfer vegetables to a tin foil-lined ovenproof tray. Roast the vegetables for 20 to 25 minutes, or until they are smooth, caramelised, and fork tender. To keep the vegetables from sticking to the grill, stir or rotate them after 10–15 min of roasting. After that, remove the pan from the heat and place it on a cooling rack.

4) Meanwhile, wash the farro in a colander over the sink after rinsing it with water. In (3L) a 3-quart saucepot, combine the Almond Breeze and farro. Add a sprinkle of salt & drizzle of olive oil to taste. To prevent spilling, bring the liquid to a boil over medium-high heat and then reduce to a gentle simmer. Cook the farro for 20 min with the lid cocked to one side to enable steam to

escape. Remove the pot from the fire but keep it on the stovetop and cover the seal. Steam for an additional 5 mins in the pot when farro is soft yet somewhat chewy in the middle. Fluff with a fork after removing the cap.

5) Combine the cooked farro and vegetables in a big serving dish & gently toss to combine until ready to serve. Combine the olive oil and balsamic vinegar in a mixing bowl and drizzle over farro salad. Toss to coat, then season to taste with salt and pepper. Serve with a squeeze of lemon and new cilantro on top. Heat the dish before serving.

4. Quinoa and Millet Mediterranean Salad

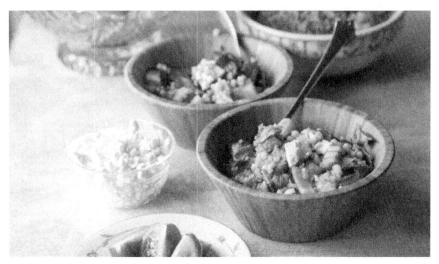

Prep Time	40 mins
Serves	3 – 4 persons

NUTRITION INFO

Calories: 641	
Calories from Fat 231 g	36 %
Total Fat 25.7 g	39 %
Saturated Fat 11.1 g	55 %
Cholesterol 59.3 mg	19 %
Sodium 764.6 mg	31 %
Total Carbohydrate 78.6 g	26 %
Dietary Fiber 12.6 g	50 %

Sugars 9.1 g	36 %
Protein 27.6 g	55 %

INGREDIENTS

- 1 cup of water
- ½ cup of millet
- ½ cup of quinoa (white, black or red)
- ¾ cup of water
- 1 English diced cucumber
- 1 diced tomato with ripe seeds squeezed out
- ½ sliced thinly red onion
- 1 pressed garlic clove
- 1 diced pepper, seeded
- 200 g diced feta cheese
- ¼ tbsp cayenne pepper
- 1 (10 ounce) drained white beans
- 2 tbsp dried dill (oregano or sub basil)
- 1 tbsp olive oil
- ¼ cup of pine nuts
- 1 lemon juice of zest as well
- Fresh ground pepper

INSTRUCTIONS

1) Bring 1 cup of water and millet to a boil, then reduce to low heat and continue to cook for five minutes. Remove from heat, cover, and set aside for ten minutes.

2) Bring 3/4 cup of water and quinoa to a boil, then reduce to low heat and cover and cook for 12-14 minutes, fluffing occasionally.

3) Toss both of the ingredients together and relax. Have fun.

5. Avocado or Shrimp/Prawn and Salad

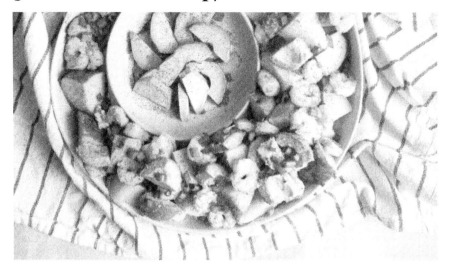

Prep Time	30 mins
Serves	2 persons

NUTRITION INFO

Calories: 435.6	
Calories from Fat 207 g	48 %
Total Fat 23 g	35 %
Saturated Fat 3.3 g	16 %
Cholesterol 157.5 mg	52 %
Sodium 727.3 mg	30 %
Total Carbohydrate 37.9 g	12 %
Dietary Fiber 10.8 g	43 %

Sugars 2.2 g	8 %
Protein 23.1 g	46 %

INGREDIENTS

- 300 g potatoes (chats 10 oz halved)
- 250 g of king prawns (cooked & peeled, 8 oz)
- 1 tbsp olive oil
- 1 minced garlic clove
- 2 sliced spring onions
- 2 tbsp Cajun seasoning
- 1 peeled, diced & stoned avocado
- salt for boil potatoes
- 1 cup alfalfa sprout

INSTRUCTIONS

1) Cook fresh potatoes for 10 to 15 minutes, or until soft, in a big saucepan of finely salted boiling water. Rinse well.

2) In a wok or big non-stick frying skillet/ pan, heat the oil.

3) Stir in the prawns, spring onions, garlic and Cajun seasoning until the prawns are hot, around 2 to 3 minutes.

4) Cook for another minute after adding the potatoes.

5) Move to serve dishes & garnish with avocado and alfalfa sprouts until serving.

6. Cobb Salad with Derby Dressing

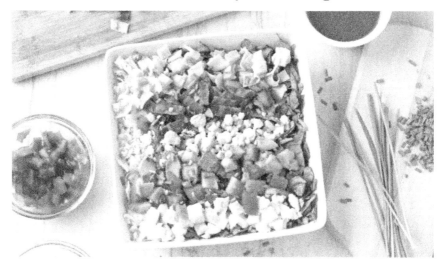

Prep Time	30 mins
Serves	2 persons

NUTRITION INFO

Calories: 832.4	0%
Calories from Fat 510 g	61 %
Total Fat 56.7 g	87 %
Saturated Fat 16.1 g	80 %
Cholesterol 352.4 mg	117 %
Sodium 3360.1 mg	140 %
Total Carbohydrate 31.2 g	10 %
Dietary Fiber 13.5 g	53 %

Sugars 12.4 g	49 %
Protein 55 g	109 %

INGREDIENTS

- ½ head of iceberg lettuce

- 1 bunch of chicory lettuce

- ½ bunch of watercress

- ½ head romaine lettuce

- ½ lb of turkey breast

- 2 skinned and seeded tomatoes

- 6 slices crisp bacon

- 1 half sliced, seeded & peeled avocado

- 3 hardboiled egg

- 2 tbsp of chopped fine chives

- ½ cup of blue crumbled cheese

INSTRUCTIONS

1) Finely chop both of the greens (almost minced).

2) In a chilled salad bowl, arrange in rows.

3) Round the tomatoes in two, remove the seeds, and chop finely.

4) The ham, tomato, eggs, and bacon can all be finely diced.

5) Arrange all of the ingredients in rows around the lettuces, plus the blue cheese.

6) Lastly, include the chives.

7) Present in this manner at the table, then toss with the dressing just before serving in cooled salad bowls.

8) Serve with a side of freshly baked French bread.

TO MAKE THE DRESSING:

9) In a blender, combine all of the ingredients, excluding the olive oil, and mix until smooth.

10) Slowly drizzle in the oil when the engine is working, then thoroughly mix.

11) Keep refrigerated until ready to use.

12) Keep this dish frozen and eat it as chilled as practicable.

Chapter:18 Main Meal Recipes

1. Grilled Lemon Salmon

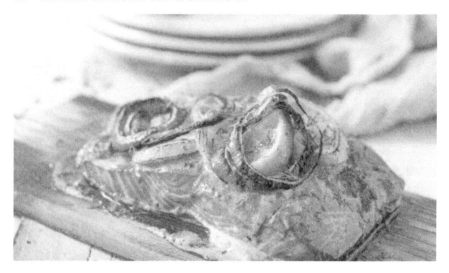

Prep Time	27 mins
Cook Time	15 mins
Serves	4 persons

NUTRITION INFO

Calories 380.7	
Calories from Fat 161 g	42 %
Total Fat 17.9 g	27 %
Saturated Fat 2.8 g	13 %
Cholesterol 78.6 mg	26 %
Sodium 1417.5 mg	59 %

Total Carbohydrate 17.3 g	5 %
Dietary Fiber 0.9 g	3 %
Sugars 14.6 g5	8 %
Protein 37 g7	4 %

INGREDIENTS

- 2 tbsp of fresh dill
- 1⁄2 tbsp of pepper
- 1⁄2 tbsp of salt
- 1⁄2 tbsp of garlic powder
- 1 1⁄2 lbs salmon fillets
- 1⁄4 cup of brown sugar
- 1 chicken mixed with bouillon cube
- 3 tbsp of water
- 3 tbsp of oil
- 3 tbsp of soy sauce
- 4 tbsp of green onions finely chopped
- 1 thinly sliced lemon
- 2 onion slices, cut into rings

INSTRUCTIONS

1) Season the salmon with dill, mustard, salt, and garlic powder.

2) Fill a small glass pan halfway with water.

3) Combine the sugar, chicken broth, soy sauce, fat, and green onions in a mixing bowl.

4) Pour the sauce over the salmon.

5) Cover and relax for 1 hour, turning halfway through.

6) Drain and toss out the marinade.

7) Place lemon & onion on top of grill on medium fire.

8) Cooked for 15 min, or until the fish is cooked through.

2. Broccoli with Garlic & Toasted Pine Nuts

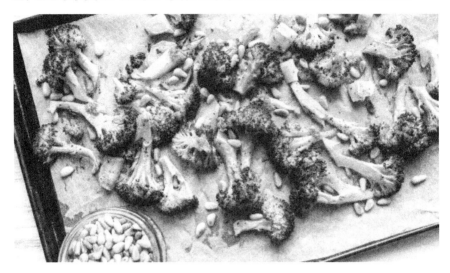

Prep Time	22 mins
Serves	4 persons

NUTRITION INFO

Calories: 172.7	
Calories from Fat 142 g	82 %
Total Fat 15.8 g	24 %
Saturated Fat 4.8 g	24 %
Cholesterol 15.3 mg	5 %
Sodium 31.8 mg	1 %
Total Carbohydrate 7 g	2 %
Dietary Fiber 0.2 g	0 %

Sugars 0.3 g	1 %
Protein 4.1 g	8 %

INGREDIENTS

- 1 lb broccoli floret
- Black pepper salt & freshly ground
- 2 tbsp olive oil
- 1 tbsp minced garlic
- 2 tbsp unsalted butter
- 1⁄2 tbsp lemon zest, grated
- 1 -2 tbsp lemon juice fresh
- 2 tbsp pine toasted nuts

INSTRUCTIONS

1) Preheat the oven to 500 degrees Fahrenheit.

2) Toss the broccoli with the oil, salt, and pepper to taste in a big mixing cup.

3) Roast the florets in a thin layer on a baking sheet for 12 minutes, or until only soft, rotating once.

4) In the meantime, melt the butter in a shallow saucepan over medium heat.

5) Heat the garlic & lemon zest for around 1 minute, stirring constantly.

6) Allow to cool slowly before adding the lemon juice.

7) Put the broccoli in a serving bowl and toss with the lemon butter to cover.

8) Sprinkle the toasted pine nuts on top.

3. Roasted Cauliflower

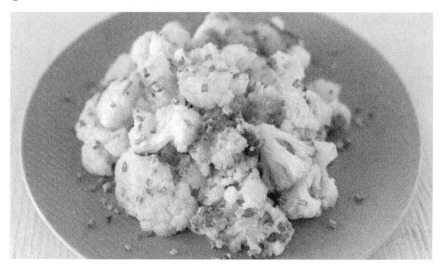

Prep Time	1 hour 10 mins
Serves	4 persons

NUTRITION INFO

Calories: 156.1	
Calories from Fat 125 g	80 %
Total Fat 13.9 g	21 %
Saturated Fat 2 g	9 %
Cholesterol 0 mg	0 %
Sodium 625.7 mg	26 %
Total Carbohydrate 7.3 g	2 %
Dietary Fiber 2.9 g	11 %

| Sugars 2.8 g | 11 % |
| Protein 2.8 g | 5 % |

INGREDIENTS

- 1 head cauliflower or an equivalent volume of commercially prepared pre-cut cauliflower
- 1 tbsp salt for taste
- 4 tbsp olive oil

INSTRUCTIONS

1) Preheat the oven to 425 degrees Fahrenheit.

2) Trim the cauliflower head, discarding the root and dense stems; split the florets into ping-pong-ball-sized sections.

3) Whisk together the olive oil and salt in a big mixing cup, then incorporate the cauliflower parts and toss well.

4) Spread the cauliflower parts on a baking sheet lined with parchment for quick cleaning (you can miss this if you don't have any), then roast for 1 hour, rotating 3 or 4 times until most of each portion has colored golden brown.

5) (The more caramelization happens and the sweeter the cauliflower parts taste, the browner they become)

6) Serve right away and enjoy.

4. Brussel Sprouts & Pan Chicken

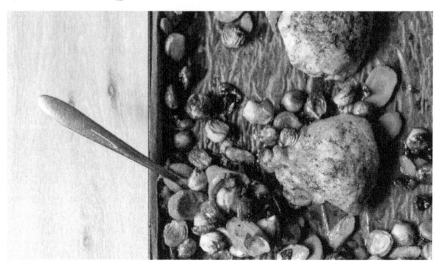

Prep Time	40 mins
Serves	4 persons

NUTRITION INFO

Calories: 323.4	0%
Calories from Fat 222 g	69 %
Total Fat 24.8 g	38 %
Saturated Fat 5.5 g	27 %
Cholesterol 79 mg	26 %
Sodium 119.9 mg	4 %
Total Carbohydrate 7.9 g	2 %
Dietary Fiber 2.5 g	9 %

Sugars 3.4 g	13 %
Protein 17.6 g	35 %

INGREDIENTS

- 4 skin on chicken thighs
- 3 tbsp of olive oil
- 1 ½ cups of halved Brussels sprouts
- 4 carrots
- 1 tbsp herbs de provence

INSTRUCTIONS

1) Preheat the oven to 400 degrees Fahrenheit.

2) Toss cut vegetables with 112 tbsp olive oil, 12 tsp herbs, and salt & pepper in a dish. Rub the vegetables all over.

3) Arrange the vegetables on a sheet tray.

4) In the same dish, position the chicken thighs. Drizzle with 112 tablespoons olive oil, 12 tablespoons spices, and season with salt and pepper. Rub the chicken all over.

5) Place the chicken in the tub.

6) Roast for 30-35 minutes, or until chicken is cooked through.

7) Switch the oven to roast AND broil for a minute or two, whether you want a crispier potato or chicken skin. If you don't keep an eye on it, it can ignite.

5. Avocado Quesadillas

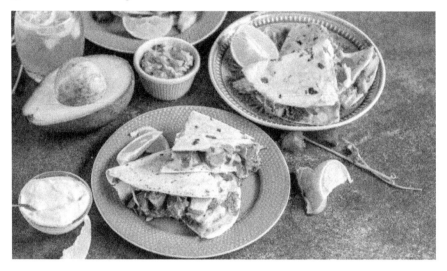

Prep Time	31 mins
Serves	2 persons

NUTRITION INFO

Calories: 794.9	
Calories from Fat 460 g	58 %
Total Fat 51.1 g	78 %
Saturated Fat 21.6 g	107 %
Cholesterol 82 mg	27 %
Sodium 978.8 mg	40 %
Total Carbohydrate 58.7 g	19 %
Dietary Fiber 11 g	43 %

Sugars 7.2 g	28 %
Protein 29.2 g	58 %

INGREDIENTS

- Salt and pepper

- 2 vine-ripe chopped seeded tomatoes into 1/4-inch pieces

- 1 tbsp chopped red onion

- 1 ripe pitted, peeled avocado & chopped into ¼-inch pieces

- ¼ tbsp of Tabasco sauce

- 2 tbsp of fresh lemon juice

- ¼ cup of sour cream

- ½ tbsp of vegetable oil

- 3 tbsp of chopped fresh coriander

- 24 inches of flour tortillas

- 1 ⅓ cups of shredded jack cheese

INSTRUCTIONS

1) Combine the avocado, tomatoes, onion, lemon juice and Tabasco in a shallow dish.

2) Season with salt & pepper to taste.

3) Mix coriander, sour cream, salt & pepper to taste in a separate little dish.

4) Brush the tops of the tortillas with oil and place them on a baking sheet.

5) 2-4 inches from the heat, broil tortillas until pale golden.

6) Sprinkle cheese thinly over tortillas and broil until melted.

7) To produce 2 quesadillas, spread the avocado mixture thinly over 2 tortillas & cover it with 1 of the leftover tortillas, cheese side down.

8) Break the quesadillas into four wedges on a cutting surface.

9) Serve warm with a dollop of the sour cream mixture on top of each wedge.

6. Club Tilapia Parmesan

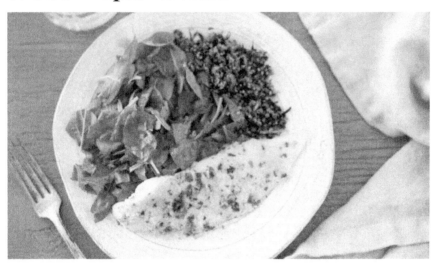

Prep Time	35 mins
Serves	4 persons

NUTRITION INFO

Calories: 376.8	
Calories from Fat 170 g	45 %
Total Fat 19 g	29 %
Saturated Fat 10.8 g	53 %
Cholesterol 155 mg	51 %
Sodium 413.3 mg	17 %
Total Carbohydrate 1.4 g	0 %
Dietary Fiber 0.2 g	0 %

Sugars 0.4 g	1 %
Protein 50.6 g	101 %

INGREDIENTS

- 2 lbs tilapia fillets

- 3 tbsp mayonnaise

- 2 tbsp lemon juice

- 4 tbsp butter, room temperature

- 1/2 cup of cheese grated parmesan

- 1/4 teaspoon of dried basil

- 3 tbsp of chopped green onions

- Black pepper

- 1/4 tbsp of seasoning salt

- 1 hot pepper sauce

INSTRUCTIONS

1) Preheat the oven to 350 degrees Fahrenheit.

2) Arrange the fillets in a single layer in a buttered baking dish or jellyroll tray.

3) Fillets cannot be stacked.

4) Lying some juice to the tip.

5) Combine the butter, cheese, onions, mayonnaise, and seasonings in a mixing dish.

6) Through a fork, thoroughly combine the ingredients.

7) Bake the fish for 10-20 minutes in a preheated oven, or until it, begins to flake.

8) Spread the cheese mixture on top and bake for 5 minutes or until golden brown.

9) The length of time it takes to bake the fish can be determined by its thickness.

10) Keep an eye on the fish to make sure it doesn't overcook.

11) This recipe serves 4 people.

12) This fish may also be cooked in the broiler.

13) 3–4 minutes under the broiler, or before nearly done.

14) Broil for another 2 or 3 minutes, just until cheese is browned.

7. Vegan Fish Fried Tacos

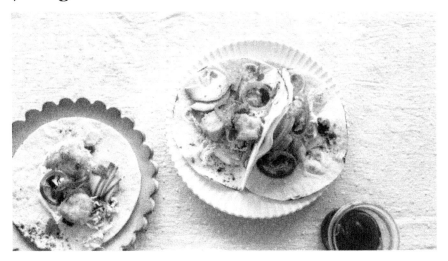

Prep Time	50 mins
Serves	2 persons

NUTRITION INFO

Calories: 378.3	
Calories from Fat 97 g	26 %
Total Fat 10.8 g	16 %
Saturated Fat 2.3 g	11 %
Cholesterol 2.1 mg	0 %
Sodium 944.8 mg	39 %
Total Carbohydrate 58.2 g	19 %
Dietary Fiber 5.7 g	22 %

Sugars 6.5 g	26 %
Protein 12.2 g	24 %

INGREDIENTS

- 14 silken tofu ounces
- 1/2 cup of plain flour
- 2 cups of panko breadcrumbs
- 1 tbsp smoked paprika
- 1/2 tbsp of salt
- 1/2 cup of milk non-dairy
- 1 tbsp of ground cumin
- 1/2 tbsp of cayenne pepper
- Vegetable oil
- 1/4 head finely shredded cabbage
- 8 tortillas
- 1 ripe of avocado

INSTRUCTIONS

1) To extract extra moisture, pat the tofu with a few bits of kitchen paper. Split the tofu into small 1-inch pieces with a knife – I want them to be small, rather than cubes, because they look better!

2) In a large shallow dish, combine the breadcrumbs.

3) In a separate large shallow dish, combine the rice, salt, smoked paprika, cayenne, and cumin.

4) In a third big shallow tub, pour the milk.

5) Toss the tofu chunks in the flour, then the milk, then the breadcrumbs, and place them on a baking sheet.

6) Fill a wide frying pan with vegetable oil to a depth of 1/2 inch. Place over medium heat and allow the oil to heat up – if a breadcrumb begins to bubble and brown, the oil is ready. Fry blocks of breaded tofu until golden beneath, then turn and finish cooking until golden all over. To drain, place on a baking sheet covered with kitchen paper. A rep for the rest of the tofu.

7) To make the pickled onion, combine the following ingredients in a small bowl.

8) In a small kettle, heat the apple cider vinegar, salt, and sugar until steaming. Pour the hot vinegar over the thinly chopped red onion in a pan or pot. Allow it to soften and transform pink for minimum of 30 minutes.

9) Serve the spicy fried tofu with pickled onion, vegan mayo, avocado, and shredded cabbage in warmed tortillas.

8. Brussels Sprouts with Onions and Bacon

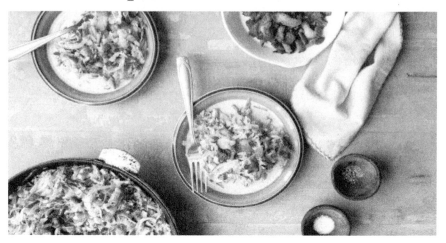

Prep Time	30 mins
Serves	4 persons

NUTRITION INFO

Calories: 45.2	
Calories from Fat 14 g	32 %
Total Fat 1.6 g	2 %
Saturated Fat 0.5 g	2 %
Cholesterol 1.8 mg	0 %
Sodium 145.9 mg	6 %
Total Carbohydrate 6.5 g	2 %
Dietary Fiber 2.2 g	8 %
Sugars 1.8 g	7 %

Protein 2.4 g	4 %

INGREDIENTS

- 2 slices OF bacon

- 1 small thinly sliced onion,

- ¼ tbsp of salt

- 1 tbsp of Dijon mustard

- ¾ cup of water

- 1 lb trimmed & thinly sliced Brussels sprout

- 1 tbsp of cider vinegar

INSTRUCTIONS

1) Cook bacon until crisp in a big skillet over medium heat (5–7 minutes); clean on paper towels, and crumble.

2) Toss the onion & salt into the drippings in the pan and fry, often stirring, unless tender & browned (about 3 minutes).

3) Scrape up any browned bits with water and mustard, then apply Brussels sprouts and fry, stirring often, until soft (4 to 6 minutes).

4) Add the vinegar and crumbled bacon on top.

Chapter: 19 Soup Recipes

1. Fresh Pea Soup

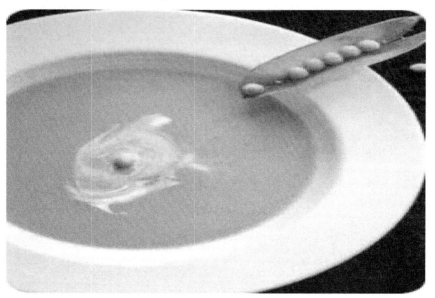

Prep Time	15 mins
Serves	2 persons

NUTRITION INFO

Calories: 172.7	
Calories from Fat 142 g	82 %
Total Fat 15.8 g	24 %
Saturated Fat 4.8 g	24 %
Cholesterol 15.3 mg	5 %

Sodium 31.8 mg	1 %
Total Carbohydrate 7 g	2 %
Dietary Fiber 0.2 g	0 %
Sugars 0.3 g	1 %
Protein 4.1 g	8 %

INGREDIENTS

- 1 piece of small diced onion
- 1 piece of minced garlic clove
- 120 grams of fresh peas
- 3 cups of vegetable stock
- 1 tsp olive oil
- 3 tbsp chopped mint
- Salt & pepper for taste

INSTRUCTIONS

1) In a saucepan, bring to a boil, then incorporate the onions and garlic. Cook for a total of 5-6 minutes.

2) Bring the stock to a simmer, and add the peas. Cook for a further 5 minutes.

3) Cook for 1-2 minutes with the lime, salt, and pepper.

4) Blend until smooth, then serve immediately.

2. Vegetarian Barley Stew

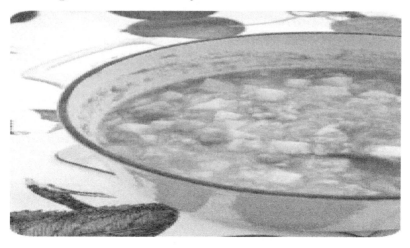

Prep Time	55 mins
Serves	3 persons

NUTRITION INFO

Calories: 641	
Calories from Fat 231 g	36 %
Total Fat 25.7 g	39 %
Saturated Fat 11.1 g	55 %
Cholesterol 59.3 mg	19 %
Sodium 764.6 mg	31 %
Total Carbohydrate 78.6 g	26 %
Dietary Fiber 12.6 g	50 %

Sugars 9.1 g	36 %
Protein 27.6 g	55 %

INGREDIENTS

- 1 diced of a small onion
- 2 cloves of minced garlic
- 1 stick of celery
- 1 washed trimmed & sliced leek
- 1 chopped carrot
- 25 grams of barley
- 1 cup water
- 25 grams of lentils
- 2 cups of vegetable stock
- 1 tbsp rosemary
- Salt & pepper for taste

INSTRUCTIONS

1) In a big saucepan, combine the stock and water before incorporating the garlic, onion, carrots, leek slices, and celery. Bring to a boil and then reduce to low heat for 10 minutes.

2) Cook for another 40 minutes after adding the barley and lentils.

3) Season to taste with salt & pepper, and top with rosemary.

3. Ramen Soup

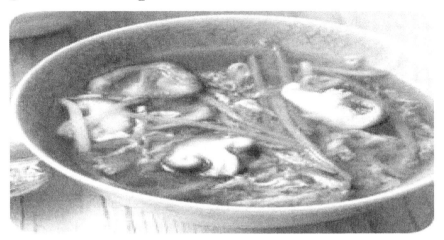

Prep Time	30 mins
Serves	2 persons

NUTRITION INFO

Calories: 376.8	
Calories from Fat 170 g	45 %
Total Fat 19 g	29 %
Saturated Fat 10.8 g	53 %
Cholesterol 155 mg	51 %
Sodium 413.3 mg	17 %
Total Carbohydrate 1.4 g	0 %

Dietary Fiber 0.2 g	0 %
Sugars 0.4 g	1 %
Protein 50.6 g	101 %

INGREDIENTS

- 1 sachet of miso soup

- 60 g of Ramen

- 40 g of shredded carrot

- 50 g of sliced thinly cabbage

- 40 g of shiitake mushroom

- Beansprouts & cilantro to garnish

- 10 g of thinly sliced chili

- 1 tsp grated ginger root

- Dash of fish sauce and soy sauce

INSTRUCTIONS

1) Cook the noodles according to the package directions.

2) To 500 mL boiling broth, add the contents of the miso soup. Next step, add the fish sauce, ginger and soy sauce.

3) Cook for an extra 1-2 minutes after adding the carrots, chili, cabbage, and mushroom.

4) Drain the noodles and drop them in the bottom of a bowl before pouring the soup on top. Serve with cilantro and beansprouts on the hand.

4. Vegetable Bean Soup

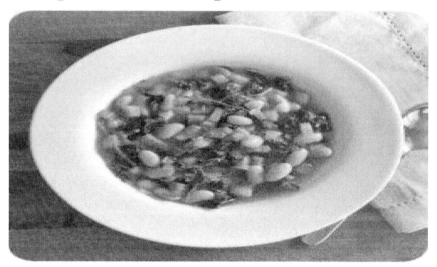

Prep Time	25 mins
Serves	2 persons

NUTRITION INFO

Calories: 123.9	0%
Calories from Fat 75 g	61 %
Total Fat 8.4 g	12 %
Saturated Fat 1.2 g	5 %
Cholesterol 0 mg	0 %
Sodium 2046.5 mg	85 %
Total Carbohydrate 11.5 g	3 %
Dietary Fiber 4 g	15 %

Sugars 5.6 g	22 %
Protein 3 g	5 %

INGREDIENTS

- 1 piece of diced onion

- 3 cloves of minced garlic

- 3 pieces of carrots

- Rinsed cannellini beans

- 1.5 L vegetable stock low-sodium

- 1 stalk of celery

- 500 g of chopped kale

- 1 tsp cumin

- 1 tsp paprika

INSTRUCTIONS

1) In a big kettle, combine all of the ingredients and bring to a boil.

2) Cook for 20 minutes before serving.

5. Chicken & Rice Soup

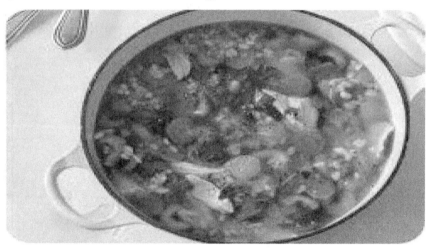

Prep Time	25 mins
Serves	3 persons

NUTRITION INFO

Calories: 832.4	0%
Calories from Fat 510 g	61 %
Total Fat 56.7 g	87 %
Saturated Fat 16.1 g	80 %
Cholesterol 352.4 mg	117 %
Sodium 3360.1 mg	140 %
Total Carbohydrate 31.2 g	10 %
Dietary Fiber 13.5 g	53 %

Sugars 12.4 g	49 %
Protein 55 g	109 %

INGREDIENTS

- ¼ tbsp of olive oil
- ½ chicken breast
- ¼ cup of onion diced
- ½ cup water
- ¼ cup of diced carrot
- ¼ cup of diced celery
- ½ cup of vegetable broth
- ½ tsp paprika
- ¼ cup of brown rice
- Handful chopped fresh herbs cilantro
- Salt & pepper for taste

INSTRUCTIONS

1) Heat olive oil in a saucepan before incorporating the celery, onion, carrot, and paprika.

2) Apply the broth & water, and also salt & pepper, after 5 minutes. Cook for 10 minutes on low heat.

3) Add the rice and new herbs to the pot with the shredded chicken breast. Cook for an extra 5 minutes before serving.

Conclusion

Before undertaking some dietary changes, even though it's only changing when you eat foods, it's still better to check with a professional healthcare practitioner. They will help you figure out if intermittent fasting is right for you. This is particularly essential for longer-term fasts that may result in vitamin and mineral deficiency. It's important to recognize that our bodies are extremely intellectual. When food is reduced at one meal, the body can experience increased hunger and calorie intake at the next meal, as well as a slowing in metabolism to match calorie consumption. While intermittent fasting has a number of possible health benefits, it cannot be believed that if strictly practiced, it would result in massive weight loss and avoid the development or worsening of the disease. It's a valuable tool, but it's possible that a combination of tools would be required to achieve and sustain optimal health.

Intermittent fasting is a lifestyle that is not only easy and healthy to follow, but it also helps to diet enjoyable. There is evidence underlying it, including the fact that it contradicts much of today's opinions and ideas. You'd imagine that with all of these fresh ideas and lifestyles, the world will be becoming more fit, rather than the obesity epidemic reaching an all-time peak. It has been shown by studies and science that IF works, and if the Romans, who were at the pinnacle of health, used it to keep in shape, why shouldn't we?

Printed in Great Britain
by Amazon